HOME EMERGENCY GUIDE

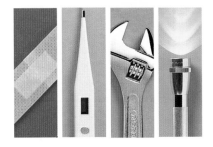

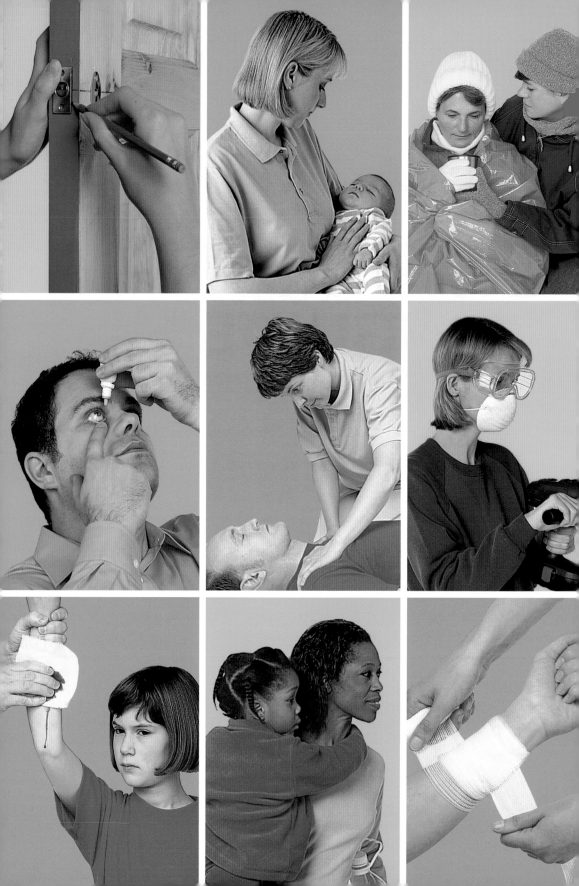

HOME EMERGENCY GUIDE

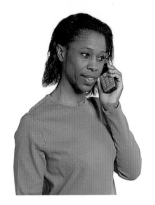

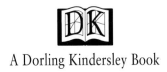

A Dorling Kindersley Book

LONDON, NEW YORK,
MUNICH, MELBOURNE, AND DELHI

CONTRIBUTORS

Dr Vivien Armstrong • Dr Sue Davidson • Professor Ian Davis
David Holloway • John McGowan • Tony Wilkins

Produced for Dorling Kindersley by
COOLING BROWN
9–11 High Street, Hampton,
Middlesex TW12 2SA

Project Editor • Alison Bolus
Senior Designer • Tish Mills
Creative Director • Arthur Brown
Managing Editor • Amanda Lebentz

DORLING KINDERSLEY
Senior Managing Editor • Jemima Dunne
Managing Art Editor • Louise Dick
Senior Art Editor • Marianne Markham
DTP Designer • Julian Dams

First published in Great Britain in 2002 by
Dorling Kindersley Limited,
80 Strand, London WC2R 0RL

A Penguin company

2 4 6 8 10 9 7 5 3

Copyright © 2002 Dorling Kindersley

A CIP catalogue record for this book is available from the British Library

ISBN 0 7513 3731 5

Colour reproduction by GRB Editrice, Verona, Italy
Printed and bound in Italy by Mondadori

See our complete catalogue at
www.dk.com

CONTENTS

1
FIRST AID

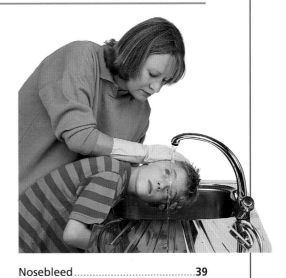

② FAMILY ILLNESS

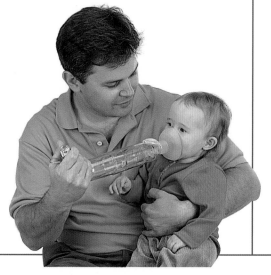

③
DOMESTIC EMERGENCIES

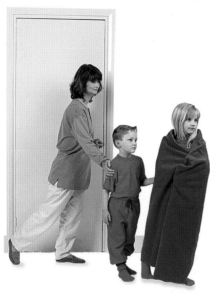

④
NATURAL DISASTERS

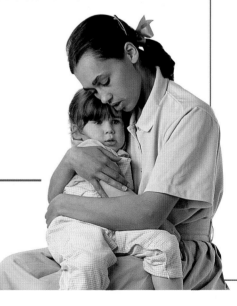

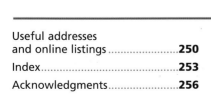

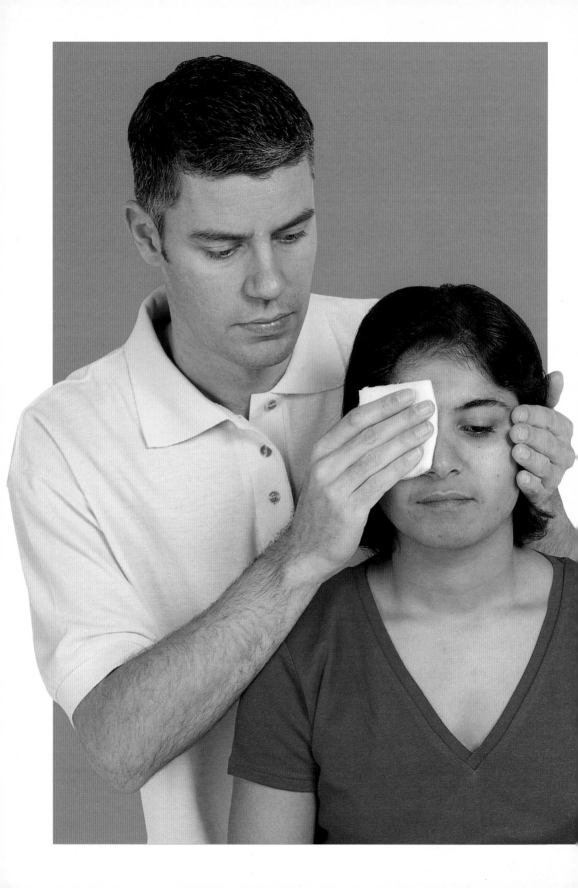

① FIRST AID

Knowing what to do in a medical emergency, such as when someone suffers a heart attack, a deep chest wound, or a snake bite, could save the casualty's life. This section tells you how to recognize important symptoms and give appropriate first-aid treatment in a wide range of situations, with full details on resuscitating an unconscious person.

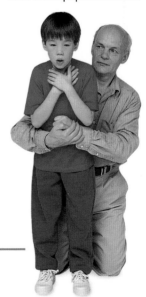

Action in an emergency

When faced with an emergency, try to remain calm and controlled so that you can act effectively. Before assessing the casualty's condition and carrying out the appropriate first aid, make sure that you are not putting yourself in danger. You will not be able to help anyone else if you become a casualty yourself. If possible, send someone for an ambulance while you deal with the situation.

ACTION PLAN

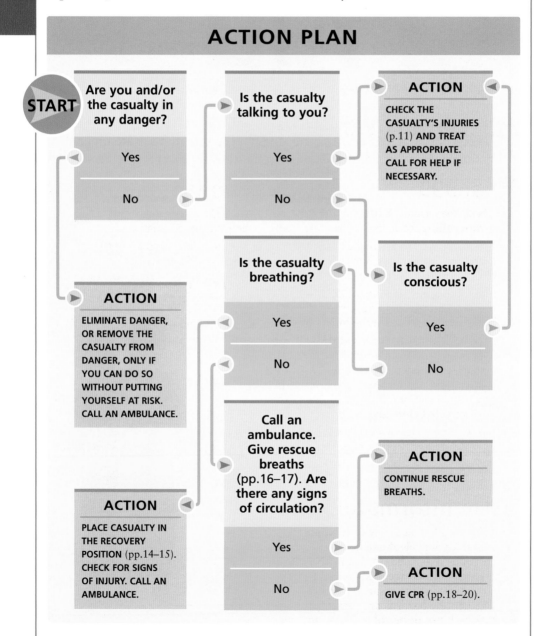

START

Are you and/or the casualty in any danger?

Yes

No

Is the casualty talking to you?

Yes

No

ACTION

CHECK THE CASUALTY'S INJURIES (p.11) AND TREAT AS APPROPRIATE. CALL FOR HELP IF NECESSARY.

ACTION

ELIMINATE DANGER, OR REMOVE THE CASUALTY FROM DANGER, ONLY IF YOU CAN DO SO WITHOUT PUTTING YOURSELF AT RISK. CALL AN AMBULANCE.

Is the casualty breathing?

Yes

No

Is the casualty conscious?

Yes

No

Call an ambulance. Give rescue breaths (pp.16–17). Are there any signs of circulation?

Yes

No

ACTION

PLACE CASUALTY IN THE RECOVERY POSITION (pp.14–15). CHECK FOR SIGNS OF INJURY. CALL AN AMBULANCE.

ACTION

CONTINUE RESCUE BREATHS.

ACTION

GIVE CPR (pp.18–20).

ASSESSING A CASUALTY'S INJURIES

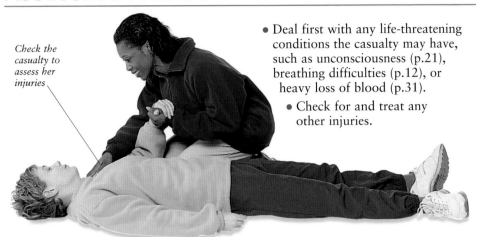

Check the casualty to assess her injuries

- Deal first with any life-threatening conditions the casualty may have, such as unconsciousness (p.21), breathing difficulties (p.12), or heavy loss of blood (p.31).
  - Check for and treat any other injuries.

CALLING AN AMBULANCE

1 Dial 999

- Check the casualty's breathing before calling for help.
- If possible, send someone else to make the call and ask him or her to confirm that help is on the way.
- If you are alone with an adult who is not breathing and you suspect a heart attack, call an ambulance.
- If you are alone with a child who is unconscious or an adult who has drowned, choked, or been injured, give rescue breaths (pp.16–17) and/or CPR (pp.18–20) for 1 minute before making the call.
- If you have to leave a casualty who is breathing, place him in the recovery position (pp.14–15).

2 Give information

- Tell the ambulance controller where you are, your telephone number, what has happened, for example a car accident, the age, sex, condition, and injuries of the casualty/ies, and whether any hazards are present, such as a fire or petrol on the road.

3 Give first aid

- Give the appropriate first-aid help to the casualty.
- Stay with the casualty until medical help arrives.
- Monitor the casualty's breathing (p.68 for an adult, p.71 for a child), pulse (p.68 for an adult, p.70 for a child), and consciousness (p.12) until the ambulance arrives.

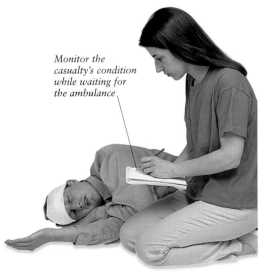

Monitor the casualty's condition while waiting for the ambulance

Resuscitation techniques

The techniques on the following pages, used in sequence, can help maintain a casualty's oxygen supply until help arrives. On finding an unconscious person, you need to open and, if necessary, clear the airway so that air can enter the lungs. If the casualty is not breathing, give rescue breaths to keep up the oxygen supply and so sustain the casualty's vital organs. If the casualty also has no circulation, give cardiopulmonary resuscitation (CPR) – rescue breaths with chest compressions – to ensure that air enters the body and is circulated by the blood. An unconscious casualty who is breathing should be placed in the recovery position, a secure position that keeps the airway open and the head, neck, and back aligned.

CHECKING FOR CONSCIOUSNESS (all ages)

1 Seek reaction

- Ask a simple question, or give a simple command, such as "Open your eyes."
- Shake an adult's shoulders gently.

! Important

- Never shake a baby or child. Instead, gently tap the shoulder or flick the sole of the foot.

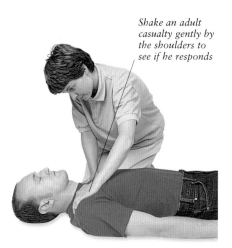

Shake an adult casualty gently by the shoulders to see if he responds

2 Assess response

- If the casualty responds to speech, assess whether he is alert and aware of the situation or muddled and sleepy.
- If he responds to touch, assess whether he reacts readily to your touch or is sluggish in response.
- If there is no reaction at all, open the casualty's airway (p.13).

3 Monitor casualty

- During first-aid treatment, you will need to repeat steps 1–2 every 10 minutes to check the casualty's level of consciousness.
- Note any changes in the casualty's responses to speech or gentle shaking (adult casualties only), and whether these indicate an improvement or a deterioration in his condition, then pass this information on to the paramedics when the ambulance arrives.
- If a conscious casualty becomes unconsciousness, open the airway (p.13), check breathing (p.14), and call for help.

OPENING THE AIRWAY (adults and children)

1 Tilt head back
- Gently place one hand on the casualty's forehead.
- Tilt the head back by pressing down on the forehead.

! Important
- If you suspect that there are head or neck injuries, handle the head carefully. Tilt the head back slightly.
- Do not sweep your fingers blindly around the mouth.

2 Remove any obstruction
- Look inside the casualty's mouth. Carefully pick out any obvious obstruction with your fingers.

3 Lift chin
- Place two fingers of the other hand under the chin and lift it gently.
- Tilt the head to open the airway. Check breathing (p.14).

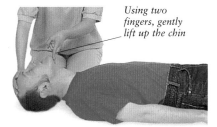

Using two fingers, gently lift up the chin

OPENING THE AIRWAY (babies under 1)

1 Tilt head back
- Place one hand on the baby's forehead then tilt the head by pressing on the forehead.

2 Remove any obstruction
- Pick out any obvious obstruction in the mouth with your fingertips.

3 Lift chin
- Place one finger of the other hand under the chin and lift it gently.
- Tilt the head slightly. If you tilt it too far, you may block the airway again. Check breathing (p.14).

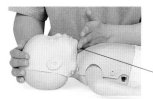

Do not over-extend the baby's neck

! Important
- Always be very gentle with a baby's head when tilting it back.

CHECKING FOR BREATHING (all ages)

2 Treat casualty

- If breathing has stopped, begin rescue breaths (pp.16–17).
- If the casualty is breathing but unconscious, place him in the recovery position (see below and opposite), then check for injuries.

1 Look for movement

- Kneel beside the casualty and put your cheek close to his mouth. Listen and feel for any signs of breathing, while looking along his chest for signs of movement.
- Do this for up to 10 seconds.

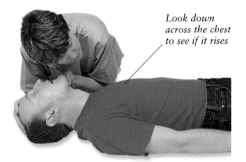

Look down across the chest to see if it rises

RECOVERY POSITION (adults and children)

2 Prepare to turn casualty

- Bring the arm farthest from you across the casualty's chest, and place the back of his hand under his near cheek.
- Pull his far leg into a bent position; keep his foot on the floor at first.
- Pull his knee towards you.

1 Position arms and legs

- Kneel alongside the casualty.
- If the casualty is wearing spectacles, remove them. Also remove any bulky objects from his pockets.
- Place the arm nearest to you so that it lies at right angles to his body, with his elbow bent at right angles and the palm of his hand facing upwards.

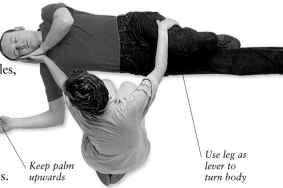

Keep palm upwards

Use leg as lever to turn body

3 Turn casualty

- Continue to pull the upper leg so that the casualty rolls on to his side. If necessary, support his body with your knees so that he does not roll too far forwards.
- Leave the casualty's hand supporting his head, and tilt the head so that the airway stays open.

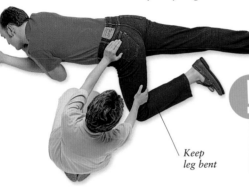

Keep leg bent

4 Support casualty

- Adjust the casualty's hand so that it supports his head. Bend the hip and knee of his upper leg at right angles so that this leg supports his body.
- Check that an ambulance is on the way.
- Check and record the casualty's breathing (p.68 for an adult, p.71 for a child), pulse (p.68 for an adult, p.70 for a child), and consciousness (p.12) until help arrives.

! Important

- If you suspect a spinal injury, do not move the casualty unless his breathing is impeded or he is in danger. Maintain his open airway.

RECOVERY POSITION (babies under 1)

BEFORE YOU START

Make sure that you have carried out the following steps:
- Checked for consciousness but had no response (p.12).
- Opened the baby's airway (p.13).
- Checked for breathing and found definite signs (see p.14).

! Important

- If you suspect a spinal injury, do not move a baby unless the breathing is impeded or he or she is in danger.

2 Monitor baby

- Monitor the baby's breathing (p.71), pulse (p.70), and level of consciousness (p.12) until help arrives.

1 Pick up baby

- Hold the baby securely in your arms so that his head is lower than his body.
- Tilt the baby's head back to keep the airway open and to allow any vomit to drain from his mouth.
- Ensure that you keep the baby's head, neck, and back aligned and supported at all times.

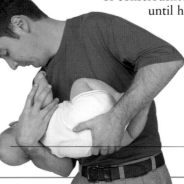

Keep the baby's head tilted downwards to let fluid drain

GIVING RESCUE BREATHS (adults and children)

BEFORE YOU START

Make sure that you have carried out the following steps:
- Checked for consciousness but had no response (p.12).
- Opened the casualty's airway (p.13).
- Checked for breathing but found no signs (p.14).

1 Breathe into casualty's mouth

- Check that the casualty's airway is still open.
- Pinch the casualty's nose closed with your thumb and index finger.
- Take a deep breath, then place your open mouth tightly around his so that you form a good seal.
- Blow air into his mouth for about 2 seconds.

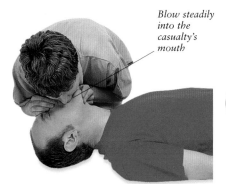

Blow steadily into the casualty's mouth

2 Watch chest

- Lift your mouth away from the casualty's mouth, keeping your hands in place to maintain his head position.
- Glance at the casualty's chest; you should see his chest fall as the air leaves his lungs. This is called an effective breath. Repeat the breath.

3 Repeat breathing

- If there is no chest movement, readjust his head and try again.
- Try rescue breaths up to five times until you achieve two effective breaths. Then check for signs of circulation (see step 4).
- If his chest still does not move, check for signs of circulation.
- If his chest does not move and you know that the casualty has choked, do not check for circulation but go straight to CPR (pp.18–20).

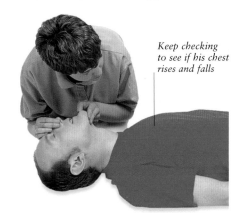

Keep checking to see if his chest rises and falls

4 Check for signs of circulation

- Look for any signs that indicate circulation – breathing, coughing, and movement of limbs – for up to 10 seconds.
- If there are signs of circulation, continue rescue breathing, giving 10 breaths per minute for adults and 20 for children. Recheck for signs of circulation every minute.
- If the casualty starts breathing again, place him in the recovery position (p.14–15).
- If there are no signs of circulation, begin CPR (pp.18–20).

Important

- If you have a face shield (p.60), use this when giving rescue breaths to prevent cross-infection.
- If the casualty has swallowed a corrosive poison, use a face shield to protect you from the effects of the chemical.
- Before giving the first breath, make sure that the casualty's head is tilted back and the airway is open.

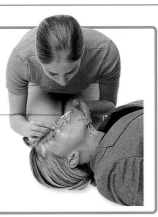

Place the shield on the casualty's face, with the filter over her mouth

GIVING RESCUE BREATHS (babies under 1)

BEFORE YOU START

Make sure that you have carried out the following steps:
- Checked for consciousness but had no response (p.12).
- Opened the baby's airway (p.13).
- Checked for breathing but found no signs (p.14).

1 Breathe into baby's mouth

- Make sure that the baby's airway is still open.
- Take a breath. Seal your lips around both the mouth and nose.
- Attempt to give one breath for about 1 second.

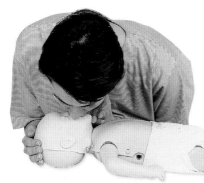

2 Watch chest

- Glance at the baby's chest; it should rise and fall. Repeat the breath.
- If the chest does not move, readjust the airway and try again.
- Try up to five times until you achieve two effective breaths. Check for signs of circulation (see step 3).
- If the chest still does not move, check for signs of circulation.
- If the chest does not move and you know the baby has choked, do not check for circulation but go straight to CPR (p.20).

3 Check circulation

- Look for any signs that indicate circulation – breathing, coughing, and movement of limbs – for up to 10 seconds.
- If circulation is present, continue rescue breathing (at a rate of one breath every 3 seconds). If there are no signs of circulation, begin CPR (p.20).

Important

- When giving rescue breaths to a baby, be careful not to blow too hard.

GIVING CPR (adults and children over 7)

1 Find compression point

- Lay the casualty on a firm surface.
- Kneel beside the casualty, level with his chest. Slide your fingers (using the hand farthest from his head) along the lowest rib to the point where it meets the breastbone.
- Position your middle and index fingers at this point.
- Place the heel of your other hand on the breastbone, just above your index finger. This is the area of the chest where you must apply the compressions.

2 Position hands

- Lift away the fingers of your first hand and lay it on top of your other hand.
- Interlock your fingers, so that the fingers of your bottom hand are not touching the chest.
- Kneel upright with your shoulders directly above the casualty and your elbows locked straight.

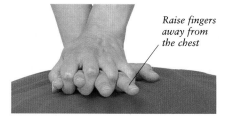

Raise fingers away from the chest

3 Compress chest

- Press downwards, depressing the breastbone by 4–5 cm (1½–2 in) in an average adult, then release the pressure but do not remove your hands from the chest.
- Compress the chest in this way 15 times at a rate of about 100 compressions per minute (roughly two every 3 seconds), maintaining an even rhythm.

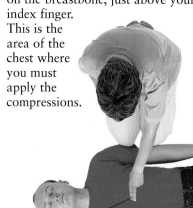

Place fingers where the lower rib and breastbone meet

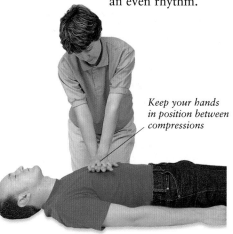

Keep your hands in position between compressions

4 Give rescue breaths

- Give the casualty two rescue breaths (p.16).

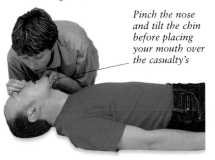

Pinch the nose and tilt the chin before placing your mouth over the casualty's

5 Repeat CPR cycles

- Continue giving cycles of 15 chest compressions and two rescue breaths until help arrives.
- If the circulation returns or the casualty starts breathing at any time, stop CPR and place him in the recovery position (pp.14–15).
- Stay with the casualty and monitor his breathing (p.68), pulse (p.68), and level of consciousness (p.12) until help arrives.

GIVING CPR (children 1–7)

BEFORE YOU START

Make sure that you have carried out the following steps:

- Checked for consciousness but had no response (p.12).
- Opened the casualty's airway (p.13).
- Checked for breathing but found no signs (p.14).
- Given two effective rescue breaths and checked for signs of circulation but found none (p.16).
- Attempted two rescue breaths and checked for signs of circulation but found none (p.16).

2 Give compressions

- Kneel upright with your shoulders directly above the child's chest and your elbow locked straight.
- Press downwards, so that you are depressing the breastbone by one-third of the depth of the chest, then release the pressure without removing your hands.
- Compress the chest five times at a rate of about 100 compressions per minute, keeping an even rhythm.
- Give one rescue breath.

1 Find compression point

- Lay the child on a firm surface.
- Find the base of the breastbone (see opposite), then position one hand on the lower half of the child's breastbone.

Position one hand ready for compressions

3 Repeat CPR cycles

- Continue giving cycles of five chest compressions to one rescue breath.
- If the child's circulation and/ or breathing return, place him in the recovery position (pp.14–15).
- Stay with the child and monitor his breathing (p.71), pulse (p.70), and level of consciousness (p.12) until help arrives.

GIVING CPR (babies under 1)

BEFORE YOU START

Make sure that you have carried out the following steps:
- Checked for consciousness but had no response (p.12).
- Opened the baby's airway (p.13).
- Checked for breathing but found no signs (p.14).
- Given two effective rescue breaths and checked for signs of circulation but found none (p.17).
- Attempted two rescue breaths and checked for signs of circulation but found none (p.17).

1 Find compression point

- Lay the baby on a firm surface.
- Position the tips of two fingers of one hand on the baby's breastbone, a finger's width below the nipples. This is the point where you must apply the compressions.

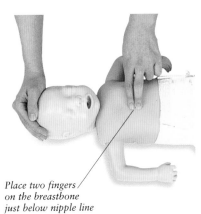

Place two fingers on the breastbone just below nipple line

! Important

- When giving rescue breaths to a baby, be careful not to blow too hard.

2 Compress chest

- Press downwards, so that you depress the breastbone by one-third of the depth of the chest, then release the pressure without moving your hands.
- Compress the chest five times at a rate of about 100 compressions per minute, keeping an even rhythm.
- Give one effective rescue breath.

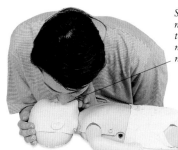

Seal your mouth over the baby's nose and mouth

3 Repeat CPR cycles

- Continue giving cycles of five chest compressions and one rescue breath.
- If the baby's circulation and/or breathing return, stop CPR and hold him in the recovery position (p.15).
- Stay with the baby and monitor his breathing (p.71), pulse (p.70), and level of consciousness (p.12) until help arrives.

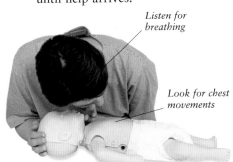

Listen for breathing

Look for chest movements

Unconsciousness

An interruption in the normal activity of the brain results in unconsciousness. This potentially life-threatening condition needs immediate medical help. The aims of first-aid treatment are to check the casualty's level of consciousness, open the airway and check breathing, then, if the casualty is breathing, to put him or her in a stable position until help arrives.

SIGNS & SYMPTOMS

- No response to loud noise or gentle shaking
- Closed eyes
- No movement or sound

TREATING UNCONSCIOUSNESS (all ages)

1 Check consciousness

- Check the casualty for signs of consciousness (p.12).
- Open the casualty's airway (p.13) and check her breathing (p.14).
- If the casualty is not breathing, begin rescue breaths (p.16 for adults and children, p.17 for babies).
- If the casualty is breathing, place her in the recovery position (pp.14–15 for adults and children, p.15 for babies) and treat any injuries (see step 3).

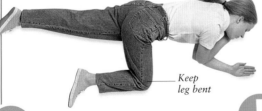

Keep leg bent

2 Summon help

- Send a helper to call an ambulance or go yourself.
- Look for clues to the cause of the condition, such as needle marks, medical warning bracelets, or cards.
- Ask bystanders for any information they may have that you can give to the emergency services.

3 Treat injuries

- Examine the casualty gently for any obvious serious injuries.
- Control any bleeding (p.31). Check for and support suspected broken arms or legs (pp.44–45).

4 Monitor casualty

- Stay with her until help arrives.
- Monitor the casualty's breathing (p.68 for an adult, p.71 for a child or baby) and pulse (p.68 for an adult, p.70 for a child or baby) every 10 minutes.
- Check for any changes in the casualty's level of consciousness by asking simple questions or shaking her gently every 5–10 minutes.

! Important

- Do not move the casualty unnecessarily in case there is spinal injury.
- If you need to leave the casualty to get help, place her in the recovery position (pp.14–15 for adults and children, p.15 for babies).
- Do not shake a baby or child.
- Be prepared to begin resuscitation (pp.12–20).
- Do not give an unconscious casualty anything to eat or drink.

Choking (adults and children)

An obstruction of the airway, usually caused by food or a foreign body, can result in choking. The aim of first-aid treatment for choking is to dislodge the object as quickly as possible. This involves encouraging the casualty to cough, then, if necessary, using back slaps and thrusts. If the obstruction is not removed, the casualty will stop breathing and lose consciousness.

SIGNS & SYMPTOMS

- Coughing, difficulty in breathing and talking
- Signs of distress, including holding the throat
- Red face and neck, later turning grey-blue

TREATING CHOKING
(adults and children over 7)

1 Encourage coughing

- Ask the casualty to cough. This may dislodge whatever is blocking the casualty's windpipe.
- Check a child's mouth to see if anything has been dislodged.

2 Give back slaps

- If the casualty is becoming weaker, bend her forwards from the waist.
- Stand slightly behind and to one side of her.
- Put one arm around her waist to support her and use your other hand to slap her sharply between the shoulder blades up to five times.
- Check the mouth again.

Keep hand flat

3 Give abdominal thrusts

- If the obstruction has still not been moved, stand behind her.
- Make a fist with one hand, place the thumb side just below her ribcage, and put the other hand on top.
- Pull upwards and inwards sharply up to five times.
- Check the mouth again.

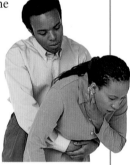

4 Repeat treatment

- If the obstruction has still not been dislodged, give three more sets of back slaps and abdominal thrusts.
- If the obstruction is still there, call an ambulance. Repeat the treatment sequence while waiting.

! Important

- If the casualty falls unconscious, open the airway, check breathing, and be prepared to begin resuscitation (pp.12–20).

TREATING CHOKING (children 1–7)

1 Encourage coughing

- If the child is still able to breathe, encourage him to cough. This may help to dislodge the obstruction.
- Check his mouth to see if anything has been dislodged. He will probably want to spit it out.

2 Give back slaps

- If the child stops coughing or cannot breathe, bend him forwards, stand or kneel behind him, and give up to five sharp back slaps between the shoulder blades.
- Check his mouth again to see if anything has been dislodged.

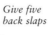

Give five back slaps

3 Give chest thrusts

- If back slaps do not help, place a fist on the lower breastbone and put your other hand over the fist.
- Pull sharply inwards and upwards up to five times.
- Check his mouth again.

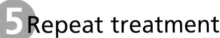

Give five sharp chest thrusts

4 Give abdominal thrusts

- If chest thrusts are not helping, move your hands down to the child's upper abdomen.
- Press sharply inwards and upwards up to five times.
- Check his mouth again.

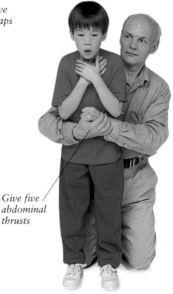

Give five abdominal thrusts

5 Repeat treatment

- If the obstruction is still there, repeat the sequence three times.
- If the obstruction has still not been dislodged, call an ambulance. Repeat the sequence while waiting.

! Important

- Do not sweep your finger around the mouth.
- If the child falls unconscious, open the airway, check breathing, and be prepared to begin resuscitation (pp.12–20).

Choking (babies under 1)

Babies under 1 can easily choke on small objects.
A choking baby may squeak, turn red then blue in the
face, and he or she may appear to cry without making
a noise. The aim of first-aid treatment is to dislodge
the object as quickly as possible, using back slaps
and chest thrusts. If the obstruction is not removed,
the baby will stop breathing and lose consciousness.

SIGNS & SYMPTOMS

- High-pitched squeak-like sounds, or no noise at all
- Difficulty in breathing
- Red face and neck, turning grey-blue

TREATING CHOKING

1 Give back slaps

- Position the baby face down along your arm, with your hand supporting her head.
- Slap her back sharply up to five times.
- Turn her over and look in her mouth to see if anything has been dislodged.
- If it has, pick it out carefully.

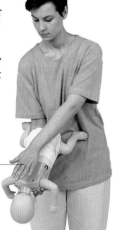

Give five back slaps

2 Give chest thrusts

- If the baby is still choking, lay her face upwards and place two fingers on her breastbone, just below nipple level.
- Push sharply into her chest with your fingers up to five times.
- Check her mouth again and remove anything that you can see.

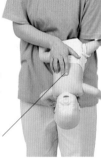

Give five sharp chest thrusts

3 Repeat treatment

- If the obstruction still has not been dislodged, repeat the sequence of back slaps and chest thrusts three more times.
- If the obstruction has not been cleared after all efforts have been made, call an ambulance.
- Take the baby with you when you go to call the ambulance.
- Repeat the treatment sequence while you are waiting for the ambulance to arrive.

! Important

- Do not blindly sweep your finger around the mouth.
- If the baby falls unconscious, open the airway, check breathing, and prepare to begin resuscitation (pp.12–20).
- Do not attempt to use abdominal thrusts on a baby.

Heart attack

A heart attack is usually caused by a blockage of the blood supply to the heart. The aims of first-aid treatment for a heart attack are to make the casualty comfortable and to arrange for transport to hospital quickly. The chances of surviving a heart attack have improved significantly in recent years, but it is still vital that the casualty is treated by medical professionals as soon as possible.

SIGNS & SYMPTOMS

- Sharp chest pain often extending down left arm
- Nausea and vomiting
- Feeling faint and breathless
- Grey skin and blueish lips
- Pulse that quickens and then weakens

TREATING A HEART ATTACK

1 Make casualty comfortable

- Raise the casualty's shoulders so that he is half-sitting and support him with cushions or pillows.
- Bend his knees and support them with more pillows.
- Give him any angina medication that he has, helping him to use it if necessary.
- Reassure him and keep him as calm as possible.

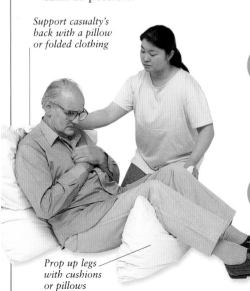

Support casualty's back with a pillow or folded clothing

Prop up legs with cushions or pillows

2 Summon help

- Call an ambulance. Tell the controller that you are with someone who is probably having a heart attack.
- Call the casualty's doctor, if you are requested to do so.

3 Give aspirin

- If any aspirin is available, give the casualty one 300mg tablet.
- Tell the casualty to chew the tablet slowly, not swallow it whole.

4 Monitor condition

- Keep the casualty calm and rested.
- Check and record the casualty's breathing (p.68), pulse (p.68), and level of consciousness (p.12) until medical help arrives.

! Important

- Do not allow the casualty to eat or drink.
- If the casualty falls unconscious, open the airway, check breathing, and be prepared to begin resuscitation (pp.12–20).

Asthma attack

During an asthma attack, muscle contractions cause the airways of the lungs to narrow, leading to the swelling and inflammation of the airways' linings. This results in difficulty in breathing, which can be life-threatening. The aims of first-aid treatment for an asthma attack are to help the casualty to breathe and to seek medical help if symptoms do not improve.

SIGNS & SYMPTOMS

- Breathing becomes difficult
- Frequent dry, wheezy cough
- Difficulty in talking
- Grey-blue tinge to skin

TREATING AN ASTHMA ATTACK

1 Calm casualty

- Sit the casualty down in a comfortable position. Leaning forwards is usually best.
- Reassure and calm her.
- Tell her to breathe slowly and deeply.

2 Provide medication

- Give the casualty her reliever inhaler (usually blue), and ask her to take a dose.
- If the casualty is a child, he or she may need to have a spacer attached to the inhaler (p.167).
- The effect of the inhaler should be obvious within minutes.

3 Repeat the dose

- If the inhaler has eased the symptoms, ask the casualty to repeat the dose.
- Encourage her to continue breathing slowly and deeply.
- Tell her to inform her doctor if the attack was unusually severe.

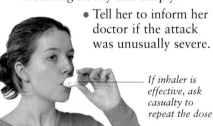

If inhaler is effective, ask casualty to repeat the dose

! Important

- Do not use a preventive inhaler (usually brown) during an attack.
- If the casualty falls unconscious, open the airway, check breathing, and be prepared to begin resuscitation (pp.12–20).

Call an ambulance if

- This is the first attack and the casualty does not have an inhaler.
- The asthma does not improve after two doses of reliever inhaler.
- The casualty is exhausted and is finding breathing increasingly difficult.

Shock

Any severe injury or illness that dramatically reduces the flow of blood around the body, such as severe bleeding or burns, can cause shock. If shock is not treated rapidly, vital organs may fail. The aims of first-aid treatment are to treat any obvious cause of shock, to improve the blood supply to the vital organs, and then to get the casualty to hospital.

SIGNS & SYMPTOMS

- Fast, then weakening, pulse
- Grey-blue tinge to lips and skin
- Sweating and cold, clammy skin
- Dizziness and weakness

TREATING SHOCK

1 Treat cause of shock

- If the cause of shock is obvious, for example severe bleeding (see p.31), treat it accordingly.

2 Make casualty comfortable

- If the casualty is breathing normally, lay him on the floor or other firm surface, on a blanket if it is cold.
- If his legs are not injured, raise and support them so that they are above the level of his heart.
- Keep the casualty still.
- Loosen any restrictive clothing around the neck, chest, and waist.
- Cover him with a blanket or coat to keep him warm if he is cold.

3 Summon help

- Call an ambulance.

4 Monitor casualty

- Monitor the casualty's breathing (p.68 for an adult, p.71 for a child or baby), pulse (p.68 for an adult, p.70 for a child or baby), and level of consciousness (p.12) every 10 minutes until help arrives.

! Important

- Stay with the casualty at all times, except if you need to call an ambulance.
- Keep the casualty still.
- Do not let the casualty eat, drink, or smoke.
- If the casualty falls unconscious, open the airway, check breathing, and be prepared to begin resuscitation (pp.12–20).

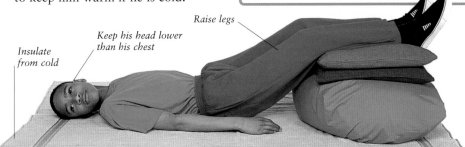

Raise legs
Keep his head lower than his chest
Insulate from cold

Anaphylactic shock

People who have developed an extreme sensitivity to a specific substance can suffer a rare and severe type of allergic reaction known as anaphylactic shock. The reaction spreads through the body, causing a sudden drop in blood pressure and narrowing of the airways, and can be fatal. The aims of first-aid treatment are to help the casualty inject epinephrine/adrenaline (Epipen) and to summon help.

SIGNS & SYMPTOMS

- Itchy red skin rash
- Swollen face, lips, and tongue
- Anxiety
- Breathing difficulties, including wheezing

TREATING ANAPHYLACTIC SHOCK

1 Summon help
- Call an ambulance, or ask someone else to do so.
- Tell the controller if you know what has caused the reaction.

2 Make casualty comfortable
- If the casualty is conscious, help him into a sitting position to ease difficulty in breathing.

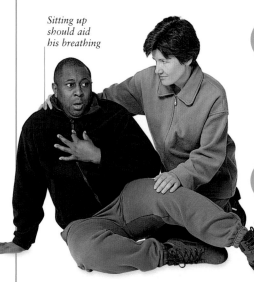

Sitting up should aid his breathing

3 Look for Epipen
- If the casualty has an Epipen, get it for him so that he can administer it.

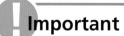

- Epinephrine, or adrenaline, is usually administered into the outer thigh, through any clothing.

Place Epipen against thigh and depress needle

4 Monitor casualty
- Monitor breathing (p.68 for an adult, p.71 for a child or baby), pulse (p.68 for an adult, p.70 for a child or baby), and level of consciousness (p.12) every 10 minutes until help arrives.

! Important
- Stay with the casualty at all times, except if you have to leave him to call an ambulance.
- If the casualty falls unconscious, open the airway, check breathing, and be prepared to begin resuscitation (pp.12–20).

Head injury

A head injury may leave no visible wound, or there may be obvious bruising or bleeding at the site. The casualty may have a headache. The aims of first-aid treatment are to control bleeding, dress the wound, and seek medical help. Even apparently minor head injuries should always be seen by a doctor.

SIGNS & SYMPTOMS

- Bleeding or bruising at site of the wound
- Depression in the skull
- Dizziness or nausea
- Headache and memory loss

TREATING A HEAD INJURY

1 Treat visible wounds

- If there is a scalp wound, replace any skin flaps.
- Press a clean pad firmly over the wound to control the blood flow.
- Keep up the pressure for at least 10 minutes until the blood flow has been stemmed.
- Secure a bandage around the casualty's head to hold the pad in position.

Lie casualty down in case of shock

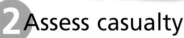

Use a pillow to support her head and shoulders

3 Monitor casualty

- Monitor breathing (p.68 for an adult, p.71 for a child or baby), pulse (p.68 for an adult, p.70 for a child or baby), and level of consciousness (p.12) every 10 minutes until help arrives.

2 Assess casualty

- Check that the casualty is fully conscious by asking simple, direct questions in a clear voice.
- If she answers your questions, lay her down in a comfortable position, then arrange for transport to hospital.
- If the casualty does not respond, ask someone to call an ambulance.
- If you need to leave an unconscious casualty to make the call yourself, place her in the recovery position first (pp.14–15).

! Important

- Use disposable gloves and/or wash your hands well when dealing with body fluids.
- If the casualty falls unconscious, open the airway, check breathing, and be prepared to begin resuscitation (pp.12–20).

Call an ambulance if

- The casualty is unconscious, appears confused, or their condition deteriorates.
- There is a depression or soft patch in the skull, or blood or watery fluid is leaking from the ears or nose; these indicate a skull fracture.

Stroke

An interruption of the blood supply to the brain, caused by a blood clot or a ruptured artery in the brain, is known as a stroke. The effect of a stroke depends on which part, and how much, of the brain is affected. Although a major stroke can be fatal, a minor stroke is not life-threatening, and a full recovery is possible. Whether the casualty is conscious or unconscious, it is important that he or she is taken to hospital as soon as possible in order to minimize any brain damage caused by the stroke.

SIGNS & SYMPTOMS

- Acute headache
- Confusion, which could be mistaken for drunkenness
- Weakness or paralysis, possibly on just one side of the body, manifested in slurred speech, drooping mouth, and a loss of limb, bladder, or bowel control
- Possible unconsciousness

TREATING A STROKE

1 Lay casualty down

- Make the casualty comfortable by laying her down and supporting her head and shoulders slightly with cushions or rolled-up blankets.
- Tilt her face to one side to allow any fluid to drain out of her mouth and wipe her face with a flannel. Alternatively, place something absorbent on her shoulder to soak up the fluid.
- Loosen restrictive clothing around her neck and chest.

2 Summon help

- Send someone to call an ambulance immediately or go yourself.

3 Monitor casualty

- Check and record the casualty's breathing (p.68), pulse (p.68), and level of consciousness (p.12) every 10 minutes until help arrives.

! Important

- Do not allow the casualty to have anything to eat or drink.
- If the casualty is or falls unconscious, open the airway, check breathing, and be prepared to begin resuscitation (pp.12–20).

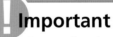

Use flannel to absorb any fluid

Severe bleeding

A heavy loss of blood is often distressing and can be life-threatening. The aims of first-aid treatment are to stop the bleeding, dress the wound as quickly as possible, and respond to any condition that may result from the heavy loss of blood or from the wound itself, such as shock or unconsciousnes.

TREATING SEVERE BLEEDING

❶ Stem blood flow

- Remove or cut away any clothing, if necessary, to expose the wound.
- Cover the injury with a sterile wound dressing, a clean pad if you have one, or with your hand.
- Press the wound firmly for 10 minutes, or longer if necessary, until the bleeding stops.
- If possible, raise the injured part above heart level. If it may also be fractured, handle it carefully.

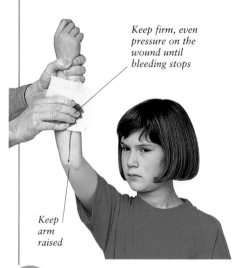

Keep firm, even pressure on the wound until bleeding stops

Keep arm raised

❷ Lay casualty down

- If the bleeding does not stop, lay the casualty on a firm surface, keeping the injury raised.
- Loosen any restrictive clothing.

❸ Secure dressing

- Bandage the wound dressing firmly but not too tightly (p.61, checking circulation).
- If blood seeps through the dressing, cover it with a second one. If bleeding continues, remove both dressings and apply a new one.

❹ Summon help

- Send someone to call an ambulance or go yourself.

❺ Monitor casualty

- Watch for signs of shock (p.27).
- Monitor breathing (p.68 for an adult, p.71 for a child or baby), pulse (p.68 for an adult, p.70 for a child or baby), and level of consciousness (p.12) every 10 minutes until help arrives.

❗ Important

- Use disposable gloves and/or wash your hands well when dealing with body fluids.
- Do not apply a tourniquet.
- If there is an object in a wound, place padding on either side of it so that the dressing will rest on the pads, not the object.
- If the casualty falls unconscious, open the airway, check breathing, and be prepared to begin resuscitation (pp.12–20).

Penetrating chest wounds

A deep wound to the chest can cause direct or indirect damage to the lungs, which may lead to a collapsed lung, and damage to the heart. The aims of first-aid treatment for a penetrating chest wound are to stop the bleeding, to help prevent the casualty from going into shock, and to get the casualty to hospital for treatment as quickly as possible.

SIGNS & SYMPTOMS

- Difficult, painful breathing
- Acute distress
- Possible presence of frothy blood at mouth
- Possible signs of shock

TREATING PENETRATING CHEST WOUNDS

1 Stem blood flow

- Expose the wound and then press against it with the palm of your hand, or get the casualty to do it himself.
- Support the casualty in a semi-upright or half-sitting position.

2 Dress wound

- Cover the wound with a sterile dressing or clean pad.
- Cover the dressing with a piece of kitchen foil, cling film, or a plastic bag to prevent air from entering the chest cavity.
- Secure the dressing with a bandage or strips of plaster or microporous tape. Apply the tape to three sides of the dressing only.

3 Make casualty comfortable

- Encourage the casualty to lean towards the side with the wound.
- Try to make him as comfortable as possible, using additional cushions or pillows to support him as necessary.
- Loosen any restrictive clothing around his waist.

4 Summon help

- Call an ambulance. Tell the controller where the injury is and describe the extent of the bleeding.
- Watch carefully for any signs of shock developing (p.27).

! Important

- Use disposable gloves and/or wash your hands well when dealing with body fluids.
- If the casualty is or falls unconscious, open the airway, check breathing, and be prepared to begin resuscitation (pp.12–20).
- If you need to put him in the recovery position (pp.14–15), lay him on his injured side.

Cover pad with cling film and secure with tape

Cuts and grazes

Small wounds, such as cuts and grazes, rarely bleed for long and require little in the way of first-aid treatment. What is important, however, is to clean the wound and apply a sterile wound dressing as quickly as possible in order to minimize the risk of infection. Check, too, that the casualty's tetanus immunization is up to date, and arrange a booster dose if necessary.

SIGNS & SYMPTOMS

- Oozing blood
- Localized pain
- Grazed area containing dirt and dust particles

TREATING CUTS AND GRAZES

1 Clean wound

- Sit the casualty down and reassure her. Even a minor fall could leave the casualty feeling shaky.
- Rinse dirt from the cut or graze under cold running water.
- Gently clean the wound and around it with sterile gauze swabs. Use a new swab for each stroke and work from the wound outwards.
- Lift any loose material, such as glass, gravel, or metal with the corner of a gauze swab.
- Carefully pat the area dry with a clean gauze swab.

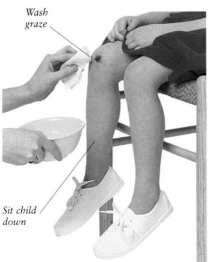

Wash graze

Sit child down

2 Dress wound

- For small cuts and grazes, cover the injury with a plaster.
- For larger injuries, place a sterile wound dressing over the affected area and hold it in place with a roller bandage (p.61).
- Rest the injured limb, preferably in a raised position.

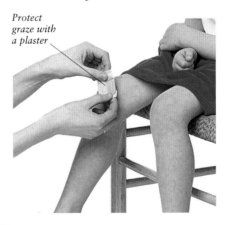

Protect graze with a plaster

! Important

- Use disposable gloves and/or wash your hands well when dealing with body fluids.
- Do not touch the cut or graze with your fingers in case you introduce an infection.
- Avoid using cotton wool or any other dry fluffy material to clean a cut or a graze – it is likely to stick to the wound.

Splinters

It is very common to find small splinters of wood embedded in the skin of the hands, knees, and feet, especially in young children. It is usually possible to remove splinters by hand or using tweezers, having made sure that the wound has been cleaned and the tweezers have been sterilized first. If splinters remain embedded or lie over a joint, seek medical help.

SIGNS & SYMPTOMS

- Fine piece of wood sticking out of skin
- Dark line under skin surface
- Blood oozing from puncture in skin

TREATING SPLINTERS

① Sterilize tweezers

- Using soap and warm water, clean the affected area thoroughly.
- Sterilize a pair of tweezers by heating them in a flame.

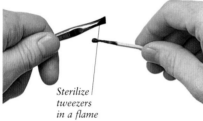

Sterilize tweezers in a flame

② Pull out splinter

- Grip the splinter with the tweezers, then pull it out in a straight line in the opposite direction to which it entered.
- Try not to break the splinter.

Grasp splinter and pull it straight out

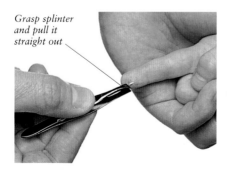

③ Clean wound

- Squeeze the area around the wound to make it bleed. This helps to flush out any remaining dirt.
- Clean the affected area and cover it with a plaster.
- Check that the casualty's tetanus immunization is up to date.

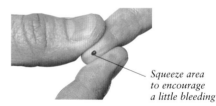

Squeeze area to encourage a little bleeding

④ Dress embedded splinter

- If the splinter breaks, or will not come out, place pads either side and bandage over it, taking care not to press down on the splinter.
- Seek medical help.

❗ Important

- Do not attempt to use a needle to lever out the splinter.
- Use disposable gloves and/or wash your hands well when dealing with body fluids.

Eye wound

Any wound to the eye is potentially serious. Blows to the eye can cause bruising or cuts, and sharp fragments of materials, such as glass, can become embedded in eye surface. Even a superficial graze can result in scarring and deteriorating vision. The aims of first-aid treatment for an eye wound are to prevent any further damage, to dress the wound, and to get the casualty to hospital.

SIGNS & SYMPTOMS

- Sharp pain in injured eye
- Visible wound or bloodshot eye
- Partial or total loss of vision
- Blood or clear fluid leaking from injured eye

TREATING AN EYE WOUND

1 Keep casualty still

- Lay the casualty on a firm surface, using a blanket if it is cold.
- Kneel down and support his head on your knees, holding it as still as possible.
- Tell him to keep both his eyes shut and still.

Tell child to keep both eyes still

Support his head

2 Dress wound

- Hold a sterile wound dressing or clean pad over the injured eye, or ask the casualty to do it, and ask him to keep his uninjured eye still.
- Keep his head steady.

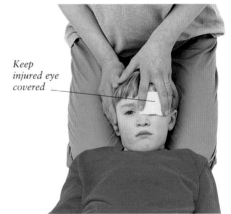

Keep injured eye covered

3 Summon help

- Ask someone to call an ambulance or call one yourself, first placing some cushions under the casualty's head to support it.
- Alternatively, if you can keep the casualty laying down and still, take him to hospital yourself.

! Important

- Do not touch the affected eye or allow the casualty to touch it.

Foreign object in the eye

Eyelashes, specks of dust, and dislodged contact lenses are common eye irritants. They usually float on the white of the eye and are easily removed. Anything that rests on the coloured part of the eye or is stuck on or embedded in the surface, however, demands hospital attention. Your aims are to prevent injury to the eye and seek hospital care, if necessary.

SIGNS & SYMPTOMS

- Pain or discomfort
- Blurred vision
- Red or watering eye

TREATING A FOREIGN OBJECT IN THE EYE

1 Examine eye

- Sit the casualty down so that she is facing the light.
- Using two fingers or your finger and thumb, gently separate the upper and lower eyelids so that you can examine the eye.

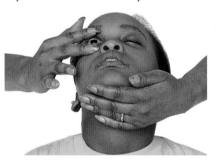

2 Flush out object

- If you can see something floating on the white of the eye or trapped under the lower lid, try to flush it out with clean water.
- Tilt the head so that the injured eye is lower than the other one.
- Pour water carefully into the corner of the injured eye, allowing it to drain away.
- Alternatively, tell the casualty to immerse her face in a sinkful of water and try blinking.

3 Lift off object

- If flushing does not work, use the corner of a clean, dampened handkerchief or tissue to lift the foreign object off the eye.
- Do not use any pressure.

4 Inspect upper eyelid

- If the object is lodged under the upper eyelid, ask the casualty to grasp the upper lashes and pull the lid over the lower one.
- If this does not help, try bathing the eye in water and asking the casualty to blink.

5 Seek medical help

- If all your efforts at removing the foreign object are unsuccessful, take the casualty to hospital.

! Important

- If anything is stuck to the eye, penetrating the eyeball, or is resting on the coloured part of the eye, treat as for an eye wound (p.35).
- Do not touch the affected eye or allow the casualty to touch it.

Chemicals in the eye

When chemicals get into the eyes, often as a result of splashing, they can cause serious damage, leading to scarring and possibly even blindness. The primary aim of first-aid treatment is to effectively irrigate the eye, or flush it with water, in order to disperse hazardous substances. The next step is to dress the eye, and then seek hospital care for the casualty.

SIGNS & SYMPTOMS

- Redness and swelling
- Watering of the eye
- Sharp pain in the eye
- Signs of chemicals nearby

TREATING CHEMICALS IN THE EYE

1 Rinse eye

- If the casualty cannot open his eye, use your finger and thumb to gently separate the two eyelids.
- Hold the affected eye under gently running cold water for at least 10 minutes.
- Be careful that water being rinsed from the injured eye does not drain into the other eye or splash either you or the casualty.
- If it is easier, use a jug or glass to pour water on to the eye.

2 Seek medical help

- Ask the casualty to hold a sterile pad, or one made from clean, non-fluffy material, such as a handkerchief, over the injured eye.
- If possible, identify the chemical.
- Take or send him to hospital.

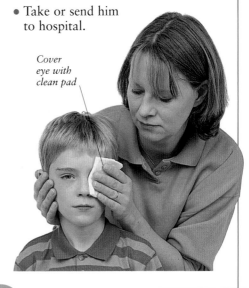

Cover eye with clean pad

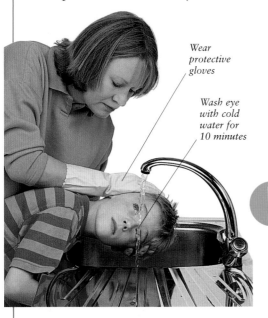

Wear protective gloves

Wash eye with cold water for 10 minutes

! Important

- Do not touch the affected eye or allow the casualty to touch it.
- If CS spray is the irritant, turn the casualty to face into the wind. Do not attempt to flush it out using water.
- Wear gloves to protect you from chemicals.

Bleeding from the mouth

Damage to a tooth and cuts to the mouth lining, lips, or tongue are common causes of bleeding from the mouth. The aim of first-aid treatment is to control severe bleeding; large amounts of blood, if swallowed, can cause vomiting, while inhalation of blood can cause choking.

TREATING BLEEDING FROM THE MOUTH

1 Control bleeding

- Ask the casualty to sit with his head forwards. This helps the blood to drain away. Give him a bowl to spit into.
- Press a gauze pad on the wound to stop the bleeding. Keep the pad in position for up to 10 minutes.

2 Monitor wound

- If the wound continues to bleed, use a fresh gauze pad and reapply pressure for a further 10 minutes.
- Encourage the casualty to spit out blood rather than swallow it.

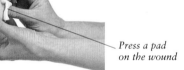

Press a pad on the wound

TREATING A KNOCKED-OUT TOOTH

1 Replant tooth

- If an adult tooth is knocked out, replant it in its socket as soon as possible and tell the casualty to see a dentist straight away.
- If you cannot replant the tooth, keep it in milk or water until the casualty reaches a dentist or doctor.
- If a milk tooth is knocked out, do not attempt to replant it.

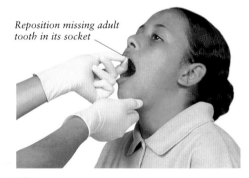

Reposition missing adult tooth in its socket

! Important

- Do not wash the mouth out, as this may disturb a clot.
- If the wound is large, or if it is still bleeding after 30 minutes of pressure, consult a dentist or doctor.

2 Control bleeding

- If the knocked-out tooth cannot be found, place a thick gauze pad across the socket, making sure that it is higher than the teeth on either side of the gap.
- Tell the casualty to bite on the pad.

Nosebleed

A nosebleed is most often caused by the rupturing of blood vessels inside the nostrils. This can happen following a blow to the nose or after sneezing or blowing the nose. Nosebleeds occur more frequently during bouts of cold or flu when the blood vessels are more fragile. The aims of first-aid treatment for a nosebleed are to control the bleeding and to comfort the casualty. A child, in particular, may find the sight and smell of the blood upsetting.

TREATING A NOSEBLEED

1 Control bleeding

- Sit the casualty down, leaning forwards, over a bowl.
- Ask her to pinch her nose just below the bridge and to breathe through her mouth. If the casualty is a child, pinch it for her.
- Tell her to avoid coughing, spitting, sniffing, swallowing, or speaking, since any of these actions could disturb a blood clot.

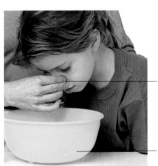

Pinch her nostrils together for 10 minutes

Let her spit into a bowl

3 Clean casualty

- When the bleeding has stopped, clean the blood away with lukewarm water, ensuring that the casualty is still leaning forwards.
- Tell the casualty to rest for a while.
- Advise her not to blow her nose as it could disturb the blood clots.

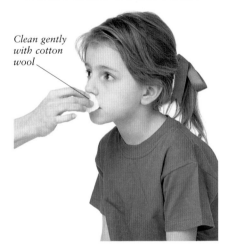

Clean gently with cotton wool

2 Assess situation

- After 10 minutes, release the pressure on the casualty's nose.
- If the bleeding continues when the pressure is released, pinch her nose for 10 more minutes.
- If, after 30 minutes, the nose is still bleeding, take or send her to hospital, still leaning forwards.

! Important

- Do not allow the casualty to lay down or tilt her head back; the blood could trickle down her throat and cause vomiting.
- If the blood is thin and watery, this indicates a fractured skull. Seek medical help immediately.

Emergency childbirth

Childbirth is rarely an emergency, since the very nature of labour means that it usually lasts for hours and therefore there is generally plenty of time to summon medical help. In the event that you do have to care for a woman who is about to give birth, however, your aims should be to keep her calm, to summon medical help, to support the mother, and to care for the baby.

TREATING EMERGENCY CHILDBIRTH

1 Summon help

- Call an ambulance, giving the name of the hospital where the mother is due to give birth, her expected delivery date, and any other relevant information.

2 Make mother comfortable

- Try to make the mother comfortable as she copes with the contractions. She may want to sit propped up, with her knees drawn up, or she may prefer to kneel, with her upper body leaning on some pillows or folded blankets. Take the lead from her as to what is best.
- Encourage her to breathe slowly and calmly during and after the contractions. Regular breathing should calm her and help with the pain; it also provides something to concentrate on.

3 Prepare equipment

- Assemble as many of the following items as possible: disposable gloves; face mask or piece of cotton material; sanitary towels; plastic bags; warm water; plastic sheeting or newspapers; clean towels; pillows; blankets.
- Wash your hands and nails thoroughly, even if you will be wearing disposable gloves.
- Put on a face mask or improvise one out of clean cotton material.
- Cover whatever surface the mother is laying on with plastic sheeting or newspapers. Add a layer of towels on top for comfort and absorbency.

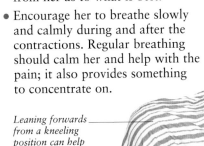

Leaning forwards from a kneeling position can help to reduce back ache

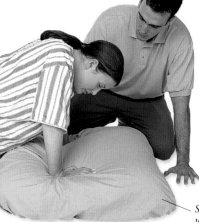

Support her with pillows

4 Monitor birth

- If the mother feels the urge to push, encourage her to bear down with each contraction.
- Tell the mother when the widest part of the baby's head is visible. At this point she needs to stop pushing and change her breathing technique to panting.
- Check for a layer of membrane over the baby's face. If there is one, tear it away.
- Check that the umbilical cord is not wrapped around the baby's neck. If it is, then very gently pull it over the head to prevent the baby from being strangled.
- Once the baby's head and shoulders are visible, the rest of the body should be expelled with the next contraction.

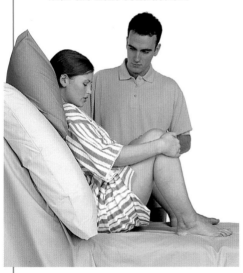

5 Check baby

- Lift up the baby very carefully and lay her on her mother's stomach.
- Newborn babies will appear blue initially. Look for signs of circulation (p.17). If the baby remains blue and shows no signs of life, begin resuscitation (pp.12–20).

6 Wrap baby

- Wrap the baby in a clean blanket or towel, still with the umbilical cord attached, and give her to the mother to hold.
- If the mother cannot hold the baby, place her on her side on a firm but soft surface.

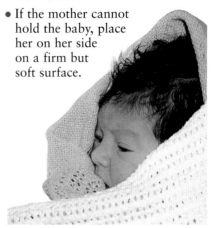

7 Deliver afterbirth

- Mild contractions will continue after the baby is born until the placenta is delivered.
- Put the placenta into a plastic bag so that a midwife or doctor can check that it is complete.
- Clean the mother with warm water and towels and give her sanitary towels to absorb any further bleeding.
- Some bleeding is normal, but if bleeding is excessive, massage the mother's stomach just below the navel to help stem the flow.
- Advise the mother to breastfeed, if possible, because it encourages the uterus to contract.

! Important

- Do not give the mother anything to eat.
- Do not pull the baby's head and shoulders out.
- Do not smack the baby.
- Do not cut the umbilical cord.
- Do not dispose of the afterbirth.

Major seizures

A convulsion, or major seizure, is the result of an electrical disturbance in the brain and consists of muscular spasms and loss of body control. Seizures that are recurrent usually indicate the brain disorder epilepsy. The aims of first-aid treatment for major seizures are to protect the casualty from injuring herself and to summon medical help if necessary.

TREATING MAJOR SEIZURES

1 Protect casualty

- If you see the casualty falling at the beginning of the seizure, try to prevent injury as she falls.
- Do not move her while she is having the seizure.
  - Loosen the clothing around her neck and try to protect her head with something soft, such as a piece of folded clothing.

Protect the casualty's head

Do not try to restrain the casualty during the seizure

2 Monitor casualty

- After the seizure, the casualty may fall into deep sleep. Check breathing (p.14), open her airway, and be prepared to resuscitate her.
- If the casualty is breathing, place in the recovery position (pp.14–15).

3 Summon help

- If the casualty remains unconscious for more than 10 minutes or convulses for more than 5 minutes, or if she has repeated seizures, call an ambulance.
- If you are not certain that the casualty is susceptible to epileptic seizures, call an ambulance.
- Monitor the casualty's breathing (p.68 for an adult, p.71 for a child or baby), pulse (p.68 for an adult, p.70 for a child or baby), and level of consciousness (p.12) until help arrives.
  - If the casualty has not had repeated seizures and you know that she has epilepsy, stay with her until she has recovered.

! Important

- Do not use force in an attempt to restrain the casualty.
- Do not put anything in the casualty's mouth.

Febrile seizures

Seizures that occur in young children as a result of a very high temperature are known as febrile seizures. Children under the age of 5 are most likely to suffer from a seizure, which is alarming to watch but is rarely dangerous to the child. Your aims are to lower the child's temperature, protect her from injury, and summon medical help.

SIGNS & SYMPTOMS

- Arched back, stiff legs and arms, and clenched fists
- Eyes rolled upwards
- Head and body jerking
- High fever

TREATING FEBRILE SEIZURES

1 Protect child

- Place pillows, rolled-up blankets, towels, or clothing around the child to help protect her from injury.
- Do not move her while she is having a seizure.

2 Cool child

- Remove clothing or bedcovers to cool the child down.
- Working from the head down, sponge the child's body all over with tepid water.
- Do not dry the child; instead, allow the moisture to evaporate from her skin.
- Do not let her get too cold.

3 Get help

- Send someone to call an ambulance or go yourself.

4 Monitor casualty

- Monitor the child's temperature at regular intervals (p.70).
- Give the recommended dose of paracetamol liquid when the seizures have stopped.
- Stop cooling her down as soon as her temperature reaches a normal 37°C (98.6°F).

! Important

- Do not use force in an attempt to restrain the child.
- Do not put anything in the child's mouth.

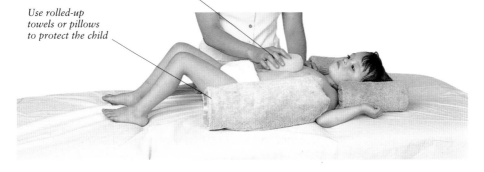

Sponge the child with tepid water until her temperature falls

Use rolled-up towels or pillows to protect the child

Broken arm

The fracture of an arm bone is not as serious as that of a leg bone (p.45) because the casualty is usually able to walk and so get to hospital relatively easily. The aims of first-aid treatment for a broken arm are to treat any bleeding, to support the injured arm with a sling, and to transport the casualty to hospital, keeping the arm as still as possible.

<table>
<tr><td>

SIGNS & SYMPTOMS

- Limb held at awkward angle
- Limb cannot be moved
- Severe pain
- Swelling and bruising
- Possible wound above fracture site

</td></tr>
</table>

TREATING A BROKEN ARM

1 Support arm

- Sit the casualty down.
- If there is a wound, treat any bleeding (p.31).
- Ask the casualty to support the injured arm across his chest so that it feels comfortable, and with the hand slightly higher than the elbow.

Keep the arm raised slightly

2 Put arm in sling

- Put some padding between the arm and the chest for comfort, then support the injured arm with a sling (p.63).
- To keep the arm still, tie another folded triangular bandage around the chest and over the sling.

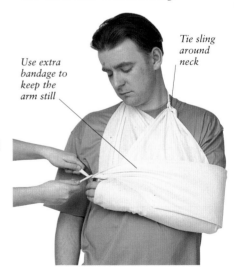

Tie sling around neck

Use extra bandage to keep the arm still

! Important

- Do not give the casualty anything to eat, drink, or smoke.
- If the elbow is injured, do not attempt to bend the arm. Lay the casualty down, surround the limb with padding, and call an ambulance.
- An injured arm may not be fractured, but if you are in doubt, treat it as a fracture until it can be X-rayed.

3 Seek medical help

- Take or send the casualty to hospital to have the arm assessed.
- Make sure that the arm is kept still on the journey to hospital.

Broken leg

The fracture of a leg bone is a serious injury that requires immediate hospital treatment. It is important that the casualty does not put any weight on the injured limb. Thigh bone fractures may involve severe internal bleeding, which can cause shock. The aims of first-aid treatment are to treat any bleeding, to support the limb, and to call an ambulance.

TREATING A BROKEN LEG

1 Support leg
- Help the casualty to lay down.
- If there is a wound, treat any bleeding (p.31).
- Put plenty of soft padding, such as rolled-up blankets or towels, on both sides of the fractured leg.
- Call an ambulance.

2 Immobilize leg
- If you can stay with the casualty, and there is no need to move her, leave the padding in place and, if necessary, support the leg with your hands.
- If you need to move the casualty out of danger, immobilize an injured leg by bandaging it to the sound one. Tie folded triangular bandages around the joints above and below the fracture site.

Hold the injured leg steady

Use a rolled-up towel to support the leg

! Important
- Do not give the casualty anything to eat, drink, or smoke.
- Do not move the casualty unless she is in danger.
- An injured leg may not be fractured, but if you are in doubt, treat it as a fracture until it can be X-rayed.

3 Monitor casualty
- Watch for signs of shock (p.27).
- Check her breathing (p.68 for an adult, p.71 for a baby or child) and pulse (p.68 for an adult, p.70 for a baby or child) while waiting for help to arrive.

Spinal injuries

Damage to the spinal cord can cause permanent loss of movement below the injured area, which means that any spinal injury is potentially serious. The aims of first-aid treatment if you suspect a spinal injury are to call an ambulance, and then keep the casualty immobile until medical help arrives, since even the slightest movement could damage the spinal cord.

SIGNS & SYMPTOMS

- Pain in neck or back
- Burning sensation or tingling in a limb
- Loss of feeling in a limb; the casualty may not be able to move his or her legs

TREATING SPINAL INJURIES

1 Summon help

- Send a helper to all an ambulance, or call one yourself.

2 Immobilize casualty

- Leave the casualty in the position in which you found her.
- Reassure her and support her head to prevent any movement.
- Ask someone to place rolled-up clothes or towels on either side of the casualty's head and body to help keep her still.
- Stay with her until help arrives.

3 Monitor casualty

- Monitor breathing (p.68 for an adult, p.71 for a child or baby), pulse (p.68 for an adult, p.70 for a child or baby), and level of consciousness (p.12) every 10 minutes while waiting for help.

! Important

- Do not move the casualty unless she is in danger or needs to be resuscitated.
- If she loses consciousness, open her airway by tilting her head only slightly, and check her breathing.
- If breathing becomes difficult, get help from several other people to place the casualty in the recovery position. Put your hands over her ears to keep her head aligned and, working as a team, roll her over very gently, making sure that you keep the neck and back aligned at all times.

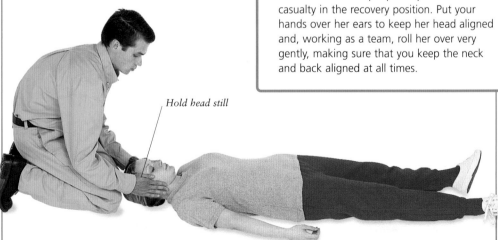

Hold head still

Sprains and strains

When ligaments and other tissues that surround and support a joint are torn or stretched, this is known as a sprain. A strain refers to muscles or tendons that are damaged or overstretched. Both injuries may lead to pain, swelling, deformity, and discoloration. Treatment follows the "RICE" procedure: rest, ice (or cold pack), compression, and elevation.

SIGNS & SYMPTOMS

- Pain and swelling in the affected area
- Deformity and discoloration

TREATING SPRAINS AND STRAINS

1 Support injury

- Steady and support the injured part.
- For extra support, place an injured limb on your knee or in your lap.

2 Cool injury

- Prepare a cold compress: either soak a flannel or towel in cold water and wring it out lightly, wrap a towel around a packet of frozen peas, or fill a plastic bag with small ice cubes. Apply the compress to the affected area to reduce swelling, bruising, and pain.
- Do not apply ice directly to the skin, because this can burn it.

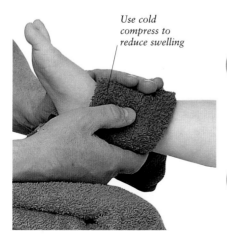

Use cold compress to reduce swelling

3 Apply compression

- Place a thick layer of padding, such as cotton wool, around the injury.
- Secure the padding in place with a roller bandage (p.62) to apply a gentle, even pressure to the injured area. Make sure that the bandage is not too tight (p.61).

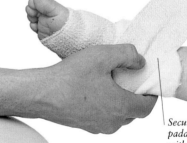

Secure padding with bandage

4 Elevate injury

- Raise and support the limb to help reduce bruising and swelling.
- Advise the casualty to rest the limb and to see a doctor.

! Important

- When you apply compression, make sure that you do not obstruct the blood supply to the tissues surrounding the injured area (p.61).

Severe burns

A burn that affects all the layers of the skin or covers a large area of the body is a severe burn. The aim of treatment is to cool down the affected area rapidly to minimize damage and loss of body fluids, and therefore reduce the risk of developing shock. Any burn larger than the palm of the casualty's hand, whatever the depth, needs hospital treatment.

SIGNS & SYMPTOMS

- Skin that is red, brown and charred, or white
- Blisters
- Possible unconsciousness
- Clear fluid weeping from skin
- Signs of shock (p.27)

TREATING SEVERE BURNS

1 Put out fire

- If the casualty's clothing is on fire, force her to the ground and use a wool or cotton blanket, rug, or coat to smother the flames (p.182).
- If possible, send someone to call an ambulance and, if necessary, the fire brigade.

2 Cool burn

- Immerse the burn in plenty of cool water, douse it with water, or cover it with cold, wet towels for at least 10 minutes.
- If there is no water, use cold milk or a canned drink to cool the burn.

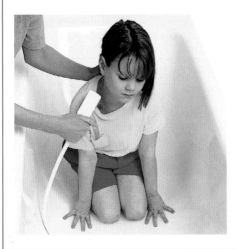

3 Expose injury

- Gently remove any clothing, belts, or jewellery near to the burn, but leave anything that is stuck to it.
- Cover the burn with a sterile wound dressing or clean non-fluffy material.

4 Make casualty comfortable

- Lay the casualty down, keeping the burn away from the ground and, if possible, above heart level.
- Call an ambulance if help is not already on the way.

5 Monitor casualty

- Monitor breathing (p.68 for an adult, p.71 for a child or baby), pulse (p.68 for an adult, p.70 for a child or baby), and level of consciousness (p.12) every 10 minutes while waiting for help.
- Watch for signs of shock (p.27).

! Important

- Do not apply any ointments to the burn.
- Do not touch the burn or burst any blisters.
- Do not put ice or iced water on the burn.

Small burns and scalds

A burn that damages only the top layer of the skin or affects a relatively small area is a small burn or scald. Although such burns can be red and painful and may swell and blister, most heal well within a few days if treated promptly. Your aims are to cool the burn and to cover it with a sterile wound dressing to minimize the risk of infection.

SIGNS & SYMPTOMS

- Red and painful skin
- Blisters weeping clear fluid

TREATING SMALL BURNS AND SCALDS

1 Cool burn

- Pour cool water over the injured area for at least 10 minutes.
- If there is no water, use cold milk or a canned drink to cool the burn.

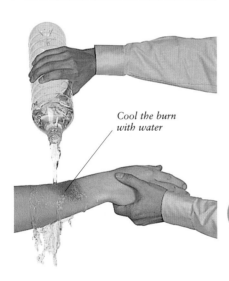

Cool the burn with water

2 Expose injury

- Gently remove any clothing, shoes, belts, or jewellery near to the burn before the area starts to swell and blister.
- Do not remove anything that is stuck to the burn because this could worsen the injury.

3 Dress burn

- Cover the burn with a sterile wound dressing or clean non-fluffy material.
- Wrap a bandage loosely over the dressing to secure it (p.61).

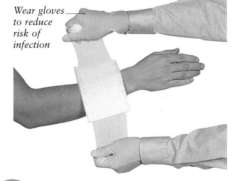

Wear gloves to reduce risk of infection

4 Monitor wound

- Check the wound daily for any signs of infection, such as pain, swelling, redness, or pus.
- If you suspect that it has become infected, advise the casualty to see a doctor at once.

! Important

- Do not apply anything other than cool liquid to the burn.
- Do not touch the burn or burst any blisters.
- Do not put ice or iced water on the burn.

Sunburn

Ultraviolet rays in sunlight can damage cells in the outer layer, causing soreness, redness, and blistering. Sunburn can occur after just 30 minutes of exposure to the sun and is most likely to occur in the middle of the day, though symptoms may take a few hours to develop. The aims of first-aid treatment are to move the casualty out of the sun, to cool the affected area, and to apply soothing lotions or creams.

SIGNS & SYMPTOMS

- Very red, hot skin
- Soreness
- Swelling
- Possible blistering
- Possible signs of heatstroke (p.52)

TREATING SUNBURN

1 Get casualty inside

- If the casualty is outside, move him into the shade or indoors.

2 Cool burn

- Get the casualty into a cold bath, or apply damp towels or cold water to the burn for at least 10 minutes.

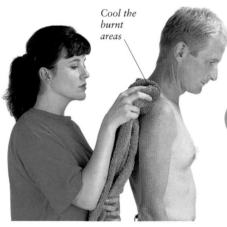

Cool the burnt areas

3 Give fluid

- See that he sips plenty of cold water while you cool his skin.

Ensure he takes small sips of fluid

4 Apply lotion

- Gently smooth calamine lotion or after-sun cream on to the burnt areas. Reapply as necessary.

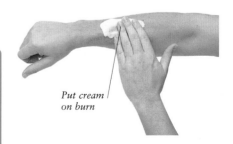

Put cream on burn

! Important

- If the skin is badly blistered, advise the casualty to see a doctor.
- If the casualty has severe sunburn and heatstroke (p.52), call an ambulance.

Heat exhaustion

Caused by excessive sweating, heat exhaustion occurs when vital salt and water are lost through the skin. People who are unused to hot and humid conditions, or those suffering from any illness that causes diarrhoea and vomiting, are often the most susceptible. The aims of first-aid treatment are to cool down the casualty and to replace lost salts and water. Heat exhaustion can develop into heatstroke.

SIGNS & SYMPTOMS

- Feeling dizzy or confused
- Headache and nausea
- Sweating, with pallid, clammy skin
- Arm, leg, or abdominal cramps
- Fast but weak pulse

TREATING HEAT EXHAUSTION

1 Make casualty comfortable

- Move the casualty to a cool place.
- Lay him down and support his legs in a raised position to improve the blood flow to vital organs.

2 Replace lost fluids

- Give him cool drinks. Ideally, offer isotonic drinks or a weak salt and sugar solution (1 teaspoon of salt and 4 teaspoons of sugar to 1 litre/ 1¾ pints of water).
- Support his head while he is drinking, if necessary.
- If he recovers, ask him to see a doctor.

3 Summon help

- If the casualty becomes weaker or confused, place him in the recovery position (p.14 for adults and children, p.15 for babies).
- Send someone to call an ambulance or go yourself.

4 Monitor casualty

- Monitor breathing (p.68 for an adult, p.71 for a child or baby), pulse (p.68 for an adult, p.70 for a child or baby), and level of consciousness (p.12) every 10 minutes until help arrives.

! Important

- If the casualty falls unconscious, open the airway, check breathing, and be prepared to begin resuscitation (pp.12–20).

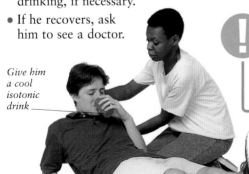

Give him a cool isotonic drink

Raise his legs

Heatstroke

If the body is exposed to high temperatures for too long, it can become dangerously overheated. The onset of heatstroke can be sudden, and the casualty may fall unconscious within a matter of minutes. The aims of first-aid treatment are to move the casualty to a cool place, to reduce his temperature, and to get him to hospital quickly.

SIGNS & SYMPTOMS

- Headache and dizziness
- Hot, flushed skin
- Poor level of response
- Rapid pulse
- Raised body temperature (over 40°C/104°F)

TREATING HEATSTROKE

1 Make casualty comfortable

- Move the casualty to a cool place.
- Remove as much of his clothing as possible.

Lay him down in cool place

Remove his clothes

2 Summon help

- Call an ambulance.

3 Cool casualty

- Drape a cold, wet sheet over the casualty. Spray or sprinkle it with water to keep it wet. Alternatively, sponge him with cold or tepid water or fan him with cold air.
- Keep cooling the casualty until his temperature drops to 38°C (100°F) under the tongue or 37.4°C (99°F) beneath the armpit (p.68 for an adult, p.70 for a child or baby).

4 Monitor casualty

- Once the casualty's temperature has fallen to 37°C (98.6°F) under the tongue or 36.5°C (97.7°F) beneath the armpit, replace the wet sheet (if used) with a dry one.
- Monitor the casualty's condition until medical help arrives.
- If his temperature rises again, cool him down following the same procedure as before.

! Important

- If the casualty falls unconscious, open the airway, check breathing, and be prepared to begin resuscitation (pp.12–20).

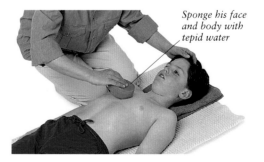

Sponge his face and body with tepid water

Fainting

Pain, fright, tiredness, hunger, emotion, or simply standing still for a long period have all been known to interrupt the flow of oxygen to the brain, which can cause a temporary loss of consciousness, or a faint. Your aims are to improve bloodflow to the casualty's brain, to make her comfortable, and to treat any injuries that may have occurred when the casualty fell. Recovery is usually rapid.

SIGNS & SYMPTOMS

- Feeling dizzy, weak, and sometimes nauseous
- Sweating
- Very pale skin
- Low pulse rate
- Brief loss of consciousness

TREATING FAINTING

1 Raise legs

- If the casualty has fainted, gently raise her legs above the level of her heart to improve blood flow.
  - If she feels faint but has not fainted, ask her to lay down, and raise her legs as for a faint.
  - Support her legs with your body or with a pile of cushions, pillows, or folded blankets.

Support legs above level of heart

2 Make casualty comfortable

- Loosen any restrictive clothing.
- Ensure that the casualty gets plenty of fresh air. If you are indoors, open a window or fan her face.
- Keep bystanders away.
- Reassure the casualty as she recovers from the fainting.

3 Treat any injuries

- Look for any injuries that the casualty may have sustained through falling.
- Treat these injuries appropriately.

4 Help casualty up

- When the casualty feels better, help her to sit up very slowly.
- If the casualty begins to feel faint again, help her to lay down.
- Raise and support her legs again, until she feels fully recovered.
- Help her to sit up again, moving very slowly and making sure that she no longer feels faint.
  - If in doubt about the casualty, call her doctor. See chart p.83 Feeling faint/passing out.

! Important

- If the casualty does not regain consciousness, open the airway, check breathing, and be prepared to begin resuscitation (pp.12–20).
- Call an ambulance.

Hypothermia

The onset of hypothermia is a reaction to exposure to cold and happens when body temperature falls below 35°C (95°F). Hypothermia may develop gradually in poorly heated houses or rapidly in freezing weather. It can also occur quickly if a body is immersed in cold water. Your aims are to warm the casualty gradually and to seek medical help if needed.

SIGNS & SYMPTOMS

- Shivering
- Cold, pallid skin
- Weak pulse
- Confusion and apathy
- Extreme tiredness

TREATING HYPOTHERMIA

1 Rewarm casualty

- Get the casualty into a shelter.
- Replace any wet clothes with warm, dry clothes and then wrap her in a survival blanket.
- If the casualty is indoors, is young and healthy, and is not lethargic or confused, help her into a warm, but not hot, bath and allow her to soak.

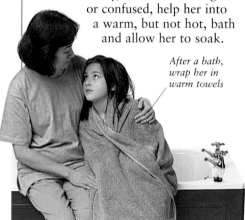

After a bath, wrap her in warm towels

2 Warm casualty in bed

- Put the casualty to bed and cover her well with blankets.
- If she is still very cold, help her put on a hat and gloves.
- Give her a warm drink to sip.

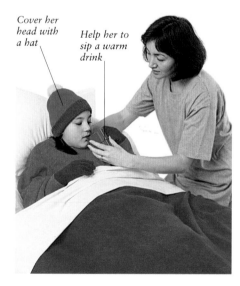

Cover her head with a hat

Help her to sip a warm drink

! Important

- Do not give the casualty alcohol to drink.
- Do not give the casualty a hot-water bottle or place her beside a fire or any other source of heat.
- If the casualty falls unconscious, open the airway, check breathing, and be prepared to begin resuscitation (pp.12–20).

3 Summon help

- If the casualty is elderly or a baby, or if her condition worries you, call a doctor.

Frostbite

In freezing conditions, especially when there is a high wind-chill factor, frostbite occurs when the body reacts to the cold by shutting down blood vessels. As a result, extremities, such as fingers and toes, may freeze and if left, these eventually become gangrenous. Hypothermia (p.54) may also occur. The aims of first-aid treatment are to rewarm the frostbitten area gradually and to seek medical help.

SIGNS & SYMPTOMS

- Sensation of pins and needles
- Pale skin becoming numb and hard
- Skin is white, mottled blue, or black

TREATING FROSTBITE

1 Warm frozen part

- Place the frostbitten part in your lap, between your hands, or get the casualty to tuck her hands into her armpits to warm them gently.
- Move the casualty out of the cold; help her if her feet are affected.
- Thaw the frostbitten part in a basin of warm water, then pat it dry.

2 Apply dressing

- Dress the affected part with a light dressing, wrapping it between frostbitten fingers and toes, and cover with a loose gauze bandage.
- Support the affected limb in a raised position to reduce the chance of swelling.

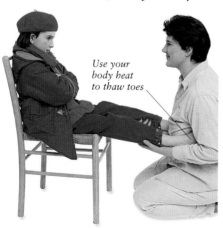

Use your body heat to thaw toes

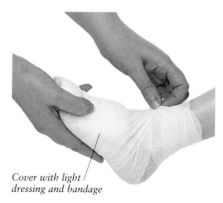

Cover with light dressing and bandage

3 Relieve pain

- As the area thaws, the skin will become hot, red, and painful.
- Give the casualty the recommended dose of paracetamol to help ease the pain.
- Take the casualty to hospital or arrange for transportation.

! Important

- Do not place a source of direct heat against the frostbitten part.
- Do not warm the frostbitten part if it may refreeze.
- Do not rub the frostbitten part.

Swallowed poisons

Poisoning can occur as a result of swallowing toxic chemicals or poisonous plants, or by overdosing on recreational or medicinal drugs. Seek immediate medical assistance and aim to provide the emergency services with as much information as possible about the poisoning, including the type of substance that was swallowed, the amount, and when.

SIGNS & SYMPTOMS

- Pain in the abdomen or chest
- Nausea, vomiting, and diarrhoea
- Breathing difficulties
- Dizziness

TREATING SWALLOWED POISONS

1 Get information

- If the casualty is conscious, ask her what poison she has swallowed.
- Look around her for signs of bottles or containers.

Ask casualty for details of poisoning

2 Summon help

- Call an ambulance.
- Tell the controller what you think the casualty has swallowed.

3 Monitor casualty

- Monitor breathing (p.68 for an adult, p.71 for a child or baby), pulse (p.68 for an adult, p.70 for a child or baby), and level of consciousness (p.12) every 10 minutes until help arrives.
- Watch for signs of deterioration.
- If alcohol poisoning is a possibility, cover the casualty with a blanket.

! Important

- Do not try to induce vomiting.
- Some poisons can cause anaphylactic shock. Look for warning signs (p.28).
- If the casualty falls unconscious, open the airway, check breathing, and be prepared to begin resuscitation (pp.12–20).
- If you need to give rescue breaths to a casualty who has swallowed a corrosive poison, protect yourself by using a face shield (see below).

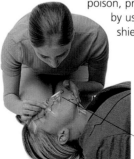

Place the shield on the casualty's face, with the filter over her mouth

Snake and spider bites

A bite from a venomous snake or spider can cause severe pain and burning at the site of the wound, with swelling and discoloration of the affected area. Most victims of such bites recover rapidly if they receive prompt hospital treatment and are given the appropriate antivenom. The aims of first-aid treatment are to seek medical assistance quickly and to try to identify the snake or spider.

SIGNS & SYMPTOMS

- Severe pain and burning
- Pair of puncture marks (snake bites)
- Nausea and vomiting
- Sweating
- Breathing difficulties
- Irregular heartbeat

TREATING SNAKE AND SPIDER BITES

1 Keep casualty still

- Lay the casualty down, keeping the heart above the level of the bite.
- Keep the casualty calm and still.

2 Clean wound

- Wash the wound carefully.
- Pat it dry with clean swabs or other non-fluffy material, but do not rub it.

3 Summon help

- Call an ambulance.
- Give the controller a description of the snake or spider that has bitten the casualty, if possible.

4 Immobilize injured part

- Place a light compression bandage on the affected part to minimize blood flow. Start bandaging just above the bite and extend up the limb.
- If a leg is affected, tie the legs together with folded triangular bandages.

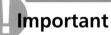
Bind legs together to immobilize injured leg

! Important

- Do not catch a venomous spider or snake to try to identify it.
- Do not apply a tourniquet.
- Do not cut the wound open or attempt to suck out the venom.

5 Monitor condition

- Monitor breathing (p.68 for an adult, p.71 for a child or baby), pulse (p.68 for an adult, p.70 for a child or baby), and level of consciousness (p.12) every 10 minutes until help arrives.

Animal and tick bites

Any animal bite carries a high risk of transmitting infection and should be seen by a doctor. Antibiotics or tetanus immunization may be required. Your aims are to stop the bleeding and clean the wound. Treating a tick bite involves removing the whole tick.

TREATING ANIMAL BITES

1 Make casualty safe

- Remove the casualty from any danger, if possible.

2 Treat severe wound

- If the wound is serious, treat as for severe bleeding (p.31).
- Take or send the casualty to hospital for urgent treatment.

3 Treat small wound

- If the wound is superficial, wash it with soap and water and pat it dry. Cover with a dressing (p.61).
- Advise the casualty to ask his doctor if immunization is needed.

! Important

- Do not try to capture the animal.
- Severe infections can be transmitted by animal bites. Seek medical advice in all cases.

TREATING TICK BITES

1 Remove tick

- Using a pair of fine-pointed tweezers, grasp the tick on either side of its body (including head and mouthparts).

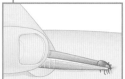

- Lever out the tick with a rocking motion.

2 Dress wound

- Wash your hands thoroughly.
- Clean the wound with antiseptic.
- Cover with an adhesive dressing.

3 Monitor casualty

- Look out for a rash at the site of the bite and/or flu-like symptoms days after the bite. In either case, send or take the casualty to a doctor in case he has developed an infection. Tell the doctor that he was bitten by a tick.

! Important

- Do not apply a hot match, alcohol, or any other substance to the tick in an attempt to remove it.
- Ensure that you remove both the head and the body of the tick.

Insect and scorpion stings

Stings from bees, wasps, and hornets are painful but are not usually life-threatening. There may be a sharp pain followed by temporary swelling, soreness, and itching. Your aims are to watch out for signs of anaphylactic shock, to remove the sting, to dress the wound, and to reduce swelling. Scorpion stings can be life-threatening and need urgent medical attention.

SIGNS & SYMPTOMS

- Sting stuck in skin
- Swollen red area
- Localized pain

TREATING STINGS IN THE SKIN

1 Remove sting

- If there is a sting in the wound, gently scrape it off with a nail or a credit card.
- Do not grasp the venom sac with your fingers or tweezers because pressure on the sac may inject more venom into the casualty.

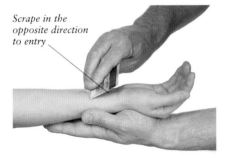

Scrape in the opposite direction to entry

2 Treat wound

- Wash the injured area with soap and water and pat dry.
- Cover the wound area with an adhesive dressing.
- Apply a cold compress on top of the adhesive dressing to reduce pain and swelling.
- Advise the casualty to seek medical help if symptoms persist.

! Important

- Call an ambulance if the casualty has been stung by a scorpion or shows signs of anaphylactic shock (p.28).

TREATING STINGS IN THE MOUTH

1 Reduce swelling

- Give the casualty a glass of cold water to sip or ice to suck, in order to reduce swelling.

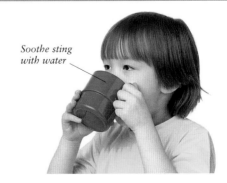

Soothe sting with water

2 Summon help

- Call an ambulance.

First-aid equipment

Having the correct supplies can make a big difference in an emergency, and you should always keep a selection of essential first-aid materials at home and in your car. Store the items in a first-aid box or in a similar type of airtight container in a dry place. The box should be easily accessible in an emergency but kept away from other medicines and out of reach of children. Ideally, the box should be small and light enough for you to carry easily. Check and replenish the first-aid kit regularly so that the contents are kept up to date.

HOME FIRST-AID KIT

ADHESIVE DRESSINGS
These are for covering small cuts and grazes

TRIANGULAR BANDAGE
This is for use as a sling to support and immobilize an injured limb

CREPE ROLLER BANDAGES
These are for applying pressure to a wound or to support a strain or sprain

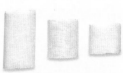

GAUZE ROLLER BANDAGES
These are for holding dressings in place on any part of the body

GAUZE DRESSINGS
These light dressings are for use directly on wounds

WOUND DRESSING
These sterile dressings combine bandage and dressing in one

Applicator

Bandage

TUBULAR BANDAGE
This is used with a special applicator to secure dressings on fingers or toes

TWEEZERS
These are for removing splinters

SCISSORS
These are for cutting dressings and bandages

ANTISEPTIC WIPES
These impregnated wipes are for cleaning wounds

ANTISEPTIC CREAM
This is spread on cuts and grazes to help prevent infection

MICROPOROUS TAPE
This breathable, low-tack tape is for holding dressings in place

SAFETY PINS
These are for securing bandages and slings

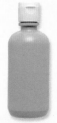

CALAMINE LOTION
This is for treating sore and sunburned skin

FACE SHIELD
This is for protection from cross-infection when giving rescue breaths

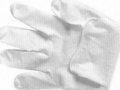

DISPOSABLE GLOVES
These are to protect against cross-infection when touching body fluids

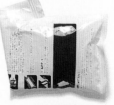

COLD PACK
This is for reducing swelling in sprains and strains

APPLYING A WOUND DRESSING

1 Apply dressing pad

- Wash your hands thoroughly and wear disposable gloves, if available.
- Choose a dressing with a pad that will cover an area 2.5 cm (1 in) beyond the edges of the wound.
- Unroll the bandage until the pad is visible, leaving a short "free" end on one side of the pad and a roll of bandage on the other.
- Place the dressing pad directly on the wound.

2 Bandage in place

- Secure the pad in place by winding the short end of the bandage once around the dressing and limb.
- Keep hold of the short end and wind the bandage roll around the dressing and limb. Continue winding the bandage until the pad is completely covered.

3 Secure bandage

- Tie the ends of the bandage together over the pad.
- Check the circulation (see below) and, if necessary, loosen the bandage and reapply.
- If blood seeps through, apply another dressing over the top. If it seeps through the second dressing, remove both and start again.

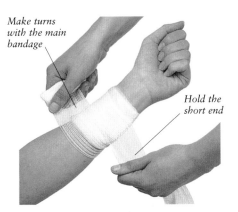

Make turns with the main bandage

Hold the short end

CHECKING CIRCULATION

1 Apply pressure

- Immediately after bandaging a limb, check the circulation in the fingers or toes beyond the bandage.
- Press on a nail or on the skin until the area turns pale, then release the pressure. The colour should return immediately.

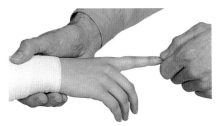

2 Loosen bandage

- If the skin colour does not return immediately, the bandage is too tight and should be loosened.
- Undo the bandage for a few turns. Wait for the colour to return to the skin, then reapply it more loosely. Check circulation again.

3 Monitor casualty

- Every 10 minutes, check fingers or toes for signs of poor circulation such as pale, cold skin, or numbness. Loosen the bandage and reapply if necessary.

APPLYING A HAND OR FOOT BANDAGE

1 Start at wrist

- Place the end of the bandage on the underside of the wrist at the base of the thumb (or ankle for a foot bandage); secure the end by making a straight turn around the wrist.
- Bring the bandage diagonally across the back of the casualty's hand in the direction of the little finger.
- Take the bandage under and across the fingers so that the upper edge touches the index finger about half way up its length.

2 Repeat layers

- Take the bandage diagonally across the back of the hand, then around the wrist and back over the hand towards the little finger.
- Continue, covering two-thirds of the previous layer with each new turn.
- When the hand is covered, make two straight turns around the wrist (or ankle) and secure the bandage.
- Check the circulation in the fingers and toes beyond the bandage (see p.61) and loosen it if necessary.

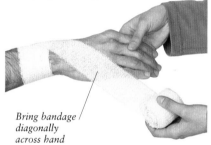

Bring bandage diagonally across hand

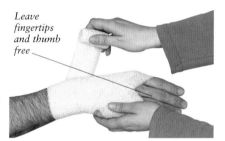

Leave fingertips and thumb free

APPLYING A TUBULAR BANDAGE

1 Apply first layer

- Cut a length of tubular gauze bandage two-and-a-half times longer than the injured finger/toe.
- Push the gauze on to the applicator then gently place the applicator over the finger.
- Hold the gauze in place at the base of the finger and pull the applicator off, leaving a layer of gauze behind.
- Hold the applicator just beyond the fingertip and twist it twice.

2 Apply second layer

- Push the applicator back over the injured finger, until the finger is covered with the rest of the gauze.
- Remove the applicator.

3 Secure bandage

- Secure the end of the gauze to the finger with a piece of adhesive tape, leaving a gap in one place.
- Make sure the bandage is not too tight. If the casualty complains of pale cold skin, numbness, or an inability to move the finger or toe, remove the bandage and hold the dressing in place by hand.

TYING AN ARM SLING

1 Support arm

- Support the arm on the injured side under the forearm or ask the casualty to support it with his other arm.
- Pass one end of the bandage under the casualty's elbow on the injured side and pull the bandage across to the opposite shoulder, so that the longest edge is parallel with his uninjured side.

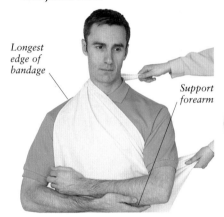

Longest edge of bandage

Support forearm

2 Form sling

- Bring the lower half of the bandage up over the forearm to meet the other end of the bandage at the shoulder on the injured side.
- Position the forearm so that the hand is slightly higher than the elbow.

Leave fingers exposed

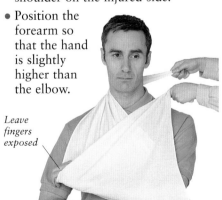

3 Secure sling

- Tie a knot at the hollow over the casualty's collarbone on the injured side of the body.
- Tuck both ends of the bandage under the knot to act as padding.

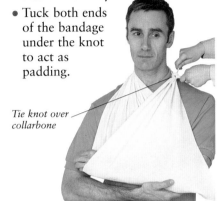

Tie knot over collarbone

4 Secure at elbow

- Fold the point of the bandage forwards at the elbow and tuck any loose bandage underneath it.
- Secure the point of the bandage to the front of the bandage with a safety pin, or twist the corner and tuck it into the sling.
- Check the circulation in the fingers after securing the sling, and again every 10 minutes (see p.61). If necessary, remove the sling and straighten the arm.

Fold point forwards

Use safety pin to secure

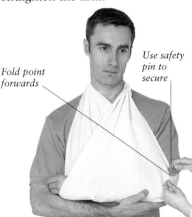

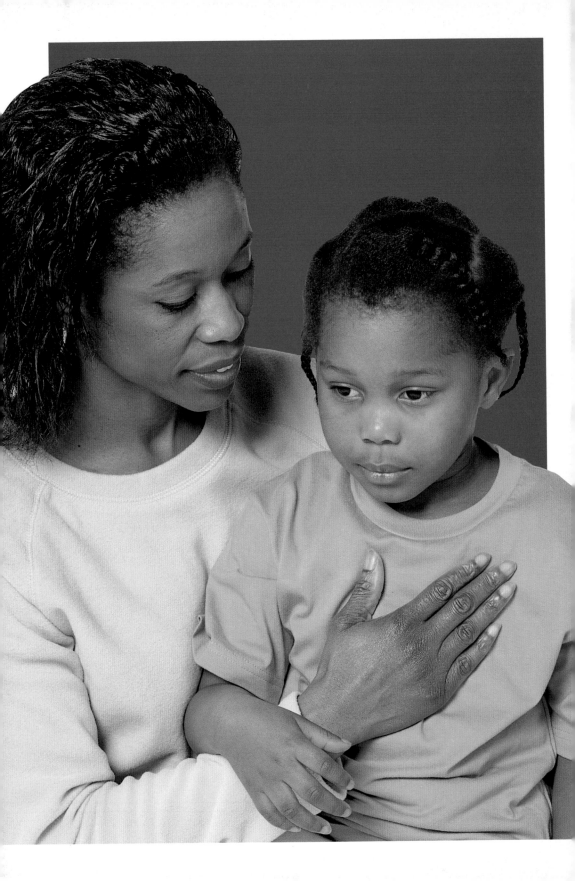

2
FAMILY ILLNESS

When a family member is ill, turn to the symptoms charts in this section to find out what is wrong. From facial pain to abdominal pain, wheezing to swollen ankles, these charts advise you on possible reasons for the symptoms and indicate how you can help.

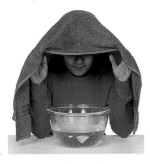

How to use this section

This section contains a selection of charts describing symptoms that may cause concern to any member of the family. At the beginning of the section there is advice on assessing for symptoms of illness, such as how to measure body temperature, take a pulse, and check breathing rates. At the end of the section there are guidelines for looking after a sick person at home, with suggestions for which medicines to keep in the home and how to administer them.

HOW TO USE THE CHARTS

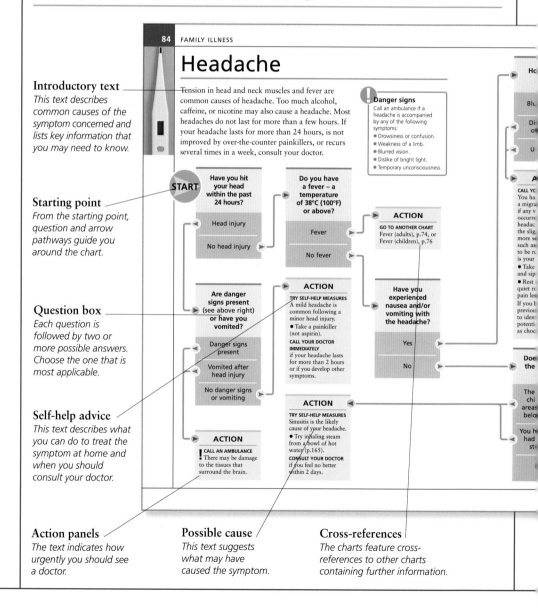

Introductory text
This text describes common causes of the symptom concerned and lists key information that you may need to know.

Starting point
From the starting point, question and arrow pathways guide you around the chart.

Question box
Each question is followed by two or more possible answers. Choose the one that is most applicable.

Self-help advice
This text describes what you can do to treat the symptom at home and when you should consult your doctor.

Action panels
The text indicates how urgently you should see a doctor.

Possible cause
This text suggests what may have caused the symptom.

Cross-references
The charts feature cross-references to other charts containing further information.

Within the chart image:

84 FAMILY ILLNESS

Headache

Tension in head and neck muscles and fever are common causes of headache. Too much alcohol, caffeine, or nicotine may also cause a headache. Most headaches do not last for more than a few hours. If your headache lasts for more than 24 hours, is not improved by over-the-counter painkillers, or recurs several times in a week, consult your doctor.

Danger signs
Call an ambulance if a headache is accompanied by any of the following symptoms:
- Drowsiness or confusion.
- Weakness of a limb.
- Blurred vision.
- Dislike of bright light.
- Temporary unconsciousness.

START → Have you hit your head within the past 24 hours?
- Head injury
- No head injury

Do you have a fever – a temperature of 38°C (100°F) or above?
- Fever
- No fever

ACTION
GO TO ANOTHER CHART
Fever (adults), p.74, or Fever (children), p.76

Are danger signs present (see above right) or have you vomited?
- Danger signs present
- Vomited after head injury
- No danger signs or vomiting

ACTION
TRY SELF-HELP MEASURES
A mild headache is common following a minor head injury.
- Take a painkiller (not aspirin).
CALL YOUR DOCTOR IMMEDIATELY
if your headache lasts for more than 2 hours or if you develop other symptoms.

Have you experienced nausea and/or vomiting with the headache?
- Yes
- No

ACTION
TRY SELF-HELP MEASURES
Sinusitis is the likely cause of your headache.
- Try inhaling steam from a bowl of hot water (p.165).
CONSULT YOUR DOCTOR
if you feel no better within 2 days.

ACTION
! CALL AN AMBULANCE
- There may be damage to the tissues that surround the brain.

SPECIAL BOXES

- Red danger signs and warning boxes alert you to situations in which emergency medical help may save a life. These boxes highlight advice that applies in particular medical circumstances.

- Blue information panels tell you how to gather the information you need to answer the questions in the chart.

Danger signs

an ambulance if a

Recurring attacks of vertigo

If you have been experiencing attacks of vertigo, it is very important to avoid certain activities that are potentially hazardous to you and to other people. You should not climb ladders or steep flights of stairs, operate machinery,

Checking a red rash

Safe alcohol limits

One unit of alcohol equals half a pint of beer, a small glass of wine or sherry, or a single measure of a spirit.

- The maximum recommended limit for men is 3 units a day.

- The maximum recommended limit for women is 2 units a day

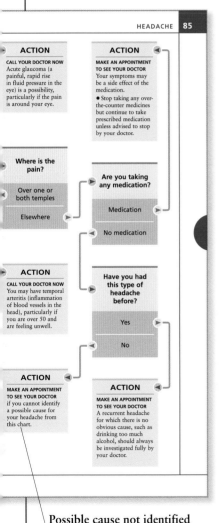

ACTION
CALL YOUR DOCTOR NOW
Acute glaucoma (a painful, rapid rise in fluid pressure in the eye) is a possibility, particularly if the pain is around your eye.

ACTION
MAKE AN APPOINTMENT TO SEE YOUR DOCTOR
Your symptoms may be a side effect of the medication.
- Stop taking any over-the-counter medicines but continue to take prescribed medication unless advised to stop by your doctor.

Where is the pain?

Over one or both temples

Elsewhere

Are you taking any medication?

Medication

No medication

ACTION
CALL YOUR DOCTOR NOW
You may have temporal arteritis (inflammation of blood vessels in the head), particularly if you are over 50 and are feeling unwell.

Have you had this type of headache before?

Yes

No

ACTION
MAKE AN APPOINTMENT TO SEE YOUR DOCTOR
if you cannot identify a possible cause for your headache from this chart.

ACTION
MAKE AN APPOINTMENT TO SEE YOUR DOCTOR
A recurrent headache for which there is no obvious cause, such as drinking too much alcohol, should always be investigated fully by your doctor.

Possible cause not identified
If your symptoms do not suggest a diagnosis, the chart recommends that you should see a doctor.

ACTION PANELS

At the end of every pathway you will find a possible diagnosis together with advice on what to do and whether or not you need to seek medical advice. There are five possible levels of attention, ranging from **CALL AN AMBULANCE**, for the most serious conditions, to **TRY SELF-HELP MEASURES**, for minor complaints. It is important to note, however, that even apparently minor complaints should receive medical attention when they occur in the elderly or in people who are undergoing cancer treatment.

! CALL AN AMBULANCE

Dial 999 for the emergency services. If there is a delay in obtaining an ambulance, go to hospital by car.

CALL YOUR DOCTOR NOW

Contact the doctor, day or night, by telephone. Dial 999 if you fail to make contact within 1 hour.

SEE YOUR DOCTOR WITHIN 24 HOURS

It is important that the symptoms are assessed by a doctor within 24 hours of their onset.

MAKE AN APPOINTMENT TO SEE YOUR DOCTOR

The condition may require medical treatment, but a reasonable delay is unlikely to lead to problems.

TRY SELF-HELP MEASURES

For minor infections, such as a sore throat or runny nose, use self-help measures, first aid, or over-the-counter remedies to relieve discomfort. Always consult your doctor if you are unsure whether a remedy is suitable and read the manufacturer's instructions before taking medication.

Assessing symptoms (adults)

Symptoms take many forms. Some involve a new sensation; others involve a change in a normal body function. Certain symptoms can be assessed very accurately because they can be measured, for example by taking a temperature or a pulse. Others need careful and regular attention to assess whether something has changed, such as breasts or testes self-examination.

MEASURING BODY TEMPERATURE

1 Insert thermometer

- Place a digital thermometer in the mouth, with the tip under the tongue, and leave it until you hear it "beep", indicating that it has measured the temperature.

2 Assess result

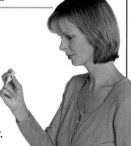

- A result above 38°C (100°F) indicates a fever.

TAKING A PULSE

1 Find pulse

- Place the pads of two fingers on the inside of a person's wrist, just below the base of the thumb.
- Press firmly to feel the throbbing beat of the pulse.
- Count the number of beats per minute.

2 Assess result

- A rate of around 72 beats per minute is normal for an adult.
  - Note the quality of the pulse: if it is regular or irregular, strong or weak.

Place the pads of the fingers below the casualty's thumb

CHECKING BREATHING RATE

1 Count breaths

- Watch for chest movement or place your hand on the adult's chest or back so you can feel the breaths.
- Count the number of breaths he or she takes in one minute.

2 Assess result

- The normal resting breathing rate is 12–15 breaths per minute.
- Note the quality of the person's breathing: if it is fast or slow, easy or laboured.

ASSESSING WEIGHT

Check whether you are a healthy weight by using the graph (right). Trace a vertical line from your height and a horizontal line from your weight. The point at which the lines cross on the graph shows your body mass index (BMI), which indicates whether or not you are within a healthy range. Being a healthy weight decreases the risk of cardiovascular disease.

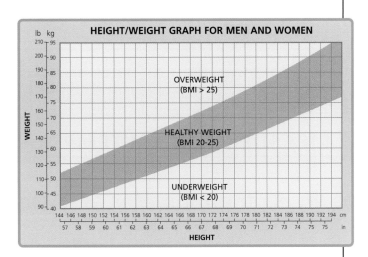

HEIGHT/WEIGHT GRAPH FOR MEN AND WOMEN

lb kg

OVERWEIGHT (BMI > 25)

HEALTHY WEIGHT (BMI 20-25)

UNDERWEIGHT (BMI < 20)

WEIGHT

HEIGHT

BREASTS: SELF-EXAMINATION

1 Examine yourself in a mirror

- The best time to examine your breasts is just after your period.
- Stand in front of a mirror and look closely for dimpled skin and any changes to your nipple or to the size or shape of your breasts.

2 Feel each breast

- Lie down with one arm behind your head and firmly press each breast in small circular movements.
- Feel around the entire breast, armpit area, and nipple.
  - If you discover a lump or any changes, consult your doctor.

Feel the breast and up into the armpit

TESTES: SELF-EXAMINATION

1 Look for changes

- The best time to examine your testes is just after a bath or shower when the scrotum is relaxed.
- Check the skin of your scrotum for changes in appearance.

2 Feel for lumps

- Feel across the entire surface of each testis by rolling each one slowly between fingers and thumb.
- Check for lumps and swellings.
- Consult your doctor immediately if you detect any change in appearance or texture.

Assessing symptoms
(children)

When a child is unwell, temperature, pulse, and breathing rate are important symptoms to assess. To monitor your child's growth, use the height and weight charts to assess whether he or she is within normal ranges.

MEASURING BODY TEMPERATURE

1 Insert thermometer

- Place a digital thermometer under the tongue (for a child over 7) or under the armpit and leave it until you hear it "beep", indicating that it has measured the temperature.
- Insert the tip of an aural thermometer into the ear. The reading is taken in 1 second.

2 Assess result

- For a mouth or ear reading, a result above 38°C (100°F) indicates a fever.
- For an armpit reading, a result above 37.4°C (99°F) indicates a fever.

Hold the digital thermometer securely in place

TAKING A PULSE

1 Find pulse

- For a baby, place two fingers on the inner side of the arm, halfway between the elbow and the armpit.
- For a child, place your fingers on the inside of the wrist, just below the base of the thumb.

2 Assess result

- Count the number of beats you can feel in one minute.
- A rate of around 140 beats per minute is normal for a baby, 120 per minute for a toddler, and 100 per minute for an older child.
- Note the quality of the pulse: if it is regular or irregular, strong or weak.

Find a pulse on the inside of the arm

CHECKING BREATHING RATE

1 Count breaths

- Place your hand on the child's chest or back so that you are able to feel the breaths.
- Count the number of breaths he or she takes in 1 minute.

Use your hand to feel how fast the baby is breathing

2 Assess result

- Compare the child's breathing rate with the maximum rate for his or her age shown in the table below.
- Note the quality of the breathing: if it is fast or slow, easy or laboured.

AGE	BREATHS PER MINUTE
Under 2 months	Maximum of 60 breaths
2–11 months	Maximum of 50 breaths
1–5 years	Maximum of 40 breaths
Over 5 years	Maximum of 30 breaths

ASSESSING HEIGHT AND WEIGHT

Find your child's age on the bottom and follow a vertical line up, then find the height or weight on the left and follow a horizontal line across. Mark the point where the lines cross. The shaded band shows the normal range of growth, and the 2nd, 50th, and 98th percentile lines indicate lower, middle, and upper limits respectively. If your child's measurements fall outside the band, see your doctor.

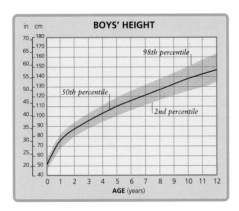

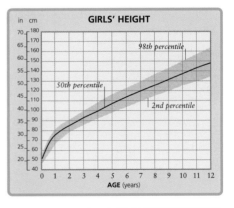

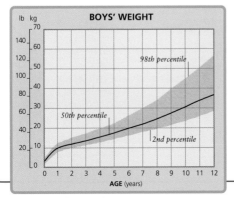

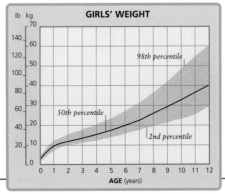

Feeling unwell

There may be times when you feel unwell without being able to pinpoint a precise symptom. This feeling is commonly caused by the onset of a minor viral illness, psychological pressures, or simply an unhealthy lifestyle. You should always consult your doctor if the feeling persists because there may be a more serious underlying problem.

START

Do you have a fever – a temperature of 38°C (100°F) or above?

Fever

No fever

Have you lost more than 4 kg (9 lb) over the past 10 weeks without changing your eating habits?

Lost over 4 kg (9 lb)

Lost under 4 kg (9 lb) or gained weight

Do you have any of the following?

Feeling constantly on edge

Difficulty sleeping

Inability to concentrate or to make decisions

None of the above

Are you taking any medication?

Medication

No medication

ACTION

GO TO ANOTHER CHART
Fever (adults), p.74 or Fever (children), p.76

ACTION

SEE YOUR DOCTOR WITHIN 24 HOURS
There are a number of possible causes for rapid weight loss, and it is important to see your doctor to rule out potentially serious conditions such as diabetes mellitus.

ACTION

MAKE AN APPOINTMENT TO SEE YOUR DOCTOR
Your symptoms may be a side effect of the medication.

● Stop taking any over-the-counter medicines but continue to take prescribed medication unless advised to stop by your doctor.

Safe alcohol limits

One unit of alcohol equals half a pint of beer, a small glass of wine or sherry, or a single measure of a spirit.

● The maximum recommended limit for men is 3 units a day.

● The maximum recommended limit for women is 2 units a day.

ACTION

MAKE AN APPOINTMENT TO SEE YOUR DOCTOR
Your symptoms may be due to an anxiety disorder or depression.
● Try physical exercise or some relaxation techniques (p.169); they may help to alleviate the symptoms.

Might you be pregnant?

Possibly pregnant

Not pregnant

Are you feeling more tired than usual?

More tired

No change

ACTION

MAKE AN APPOINTMENT TO SEE YOUR DOCTOR
if your tiredness is persistent or severe and has no obvious cause.

ACTION

TRY SELF-HELP MEASURES
Body changes that occur soon after conception can make you feel unwell. Symptoms include tiredness, feeling faint, and nausea/vomiting.
● Eat frequent small meals throughout the day rather than a few larger meals. If you suffer from morning sickness, eat a snack before getting up.
● Lie down if you are feeling faint or tired.
● If you are not sure whether you are pregnant, use a home pregnancy test or consult your doctor.

Do you regularly drink more than the recommended limit of alcohol (see box opposite)?

Within the limit

More than the limit

ACTION

MAKE AN APPOINTMENT TO SEE YOUR DOCTOR
for advice about reducing the amount of alcohol you drink. Regularly drinking too much alcohol can make you feel unwell.

ACTION

TRY SELF-HELP MEASURES
You may have a mild digestive upset as a result of infection or having eaten something that disagrees with you. Your symptoms are not likely to be dangerous, but severe diarrhoea can cause dehydration, particularly in the elderly or very young.
● Avoid rich or spicy foods and drink plenty of clear fluids.

CONSULT YOUR DOCTOR
if you do not feel better within 2 days or sooner for a child.

Do you have any of the following?

Loss of appetite

Nausea and/or vomiting

Diarrhoea

None of the above

ACTION

MAKE AN APPOINTMENT TO SEE YOUR DOCTOR
if you cannot identify a possible cause for feeling unwell from this chart.

Fever (adults)

For children under 12, see p.76 ▶

Normal temperature varies from one person to another, but if your temperature is 38°C (100°F) or above, you have a fever. Most fevers are due to infection, but heat exposure or certain drugs can also raise body temperature. In all cases, follow the advice for bringing down a fever (p.164).

! High temperature

If you are feeling unwell, you should take your temperature every 4 hours.

- Call your doctor immediately if your temperature rises to 39°C (102°F) or above.
- Take steps to lower the fever without delay (see Bringing down a fever, p.164).

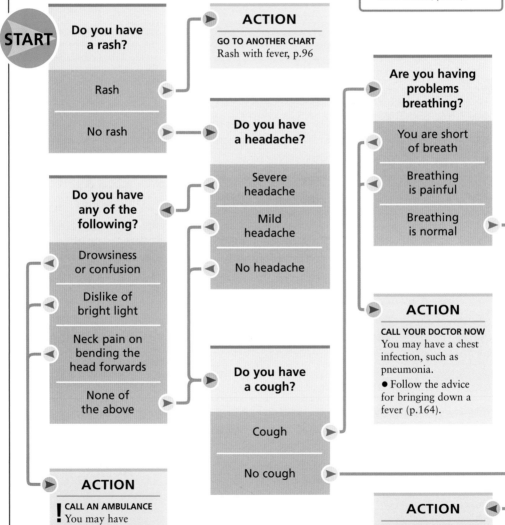

START

Do you have a rash?

Rash ▶

No rash ▶

ACTION

GO TO ANOTHER CHART
Rash with fever, p.96

Do you have a headache?

Severe headache

Mild headache

No headache

Do you have any of the following?

Drowsiness or confusion

Dislike of bright light

Neck pain on bending the head forwards

None of the above ▶

Do you have a cough?

Cough ▶

No cough ▶

Are you having problems breathing?

You are short of breath

Breathing is painful

Breathing is normal ▶

ACTION

CALL YOUR DOCTOR NOW
You may have a chest infection, such as pneumonia.

- Follow the advice for bringing down a fever (p.164).

ACTION

! CALL AN AMBULANCE
You may have meningitis (infection inflaming membranes around the brain).

ACTION

GO TO ANOTHER CHART
Sore throat, p.103

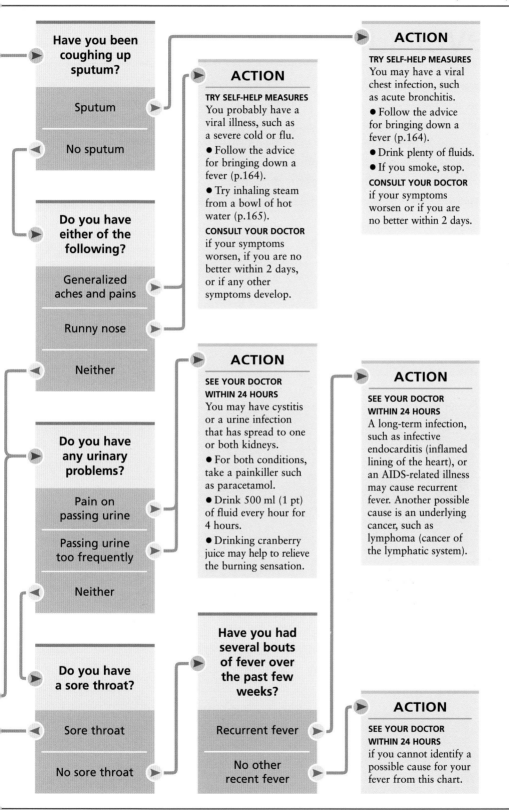

Have you been coughing up sputum?

Sputum →

No sputum →

ACTION

TRY SELF-HELP MEASURES
You probably have a viral illness, such as a severe cold or flu.
● Follow the advice for bringing down a fever (p.164).
● Try inhaling steam from a bowl of hot water (p.165).
CONSULT YOUR DOCTOR
if your symptoms worsen, if you are no better within 2 days, or if any other symptoms develop.

ACTION

TRY SELF-HELP MEASURES
You may have a viral chest infection, such as acute bronchitis.
● Follow the advice for bringing down a fever (p.164).
● Drink plenty of fluids.
● If you smoke, stop.
CONSULT YOUR DOCTOR
if your symptoms worsen or if you are no better within 2 days.

Do you have either of the following?

Generalized aches and pains →

Runny nose →

Neither →

Do you have any urinary problems?

Pain on passing urine →

Passing urine too frequently →

Neither →

ACTION

SEE YOUR DOCTOR WITHIN 24 HOURS
You may have cystitis or a urine infection that has spread to one or both kidneys.
● For both conditions, take a painkiller such as paracetamol.
● Drink 500 ml (1 pt) of fluid every hour for 4 hours.
● Drinking cranberry juice may help to relieve the burning sensation.

ACTION

SEE YOUR DOCTOR WITHIN 24 HOURS
A long-term infection, such as infective endocarditis (inflamed lining of the heart), or an AIDS-related illness may cause recurrent fever. Another possible cause is an underlying cancer, such as lymphoma (cancer of the lymphatic system).

Do you have a sore throat?

Sore throat →

No sore throat →

Have you had several bouts of fever over the past few weeks?

Recurrent fever →

No other recent fever →

ACTION

SEE YOUR DOCTOR WITHIN 24 HOURS
if you cannot identify a possible cause for your fever from this chart.

Fever (children)

◀ **For adults and children over 12, see p.74**

A fever is a temperature of 38°C (100°F) or above. If your child is unwell, you should take his or her temperature because a high fever may need urgent treatment. If a feverish child becomes unresponsive, call an ambulance. In all cases, follow the advice for bringing down a fever (p.164).

Danger signs

Call an ambulance if your child's temperature rises above 39°C (102°F) and he or she has any of the following symptoms:

● Abnormally rapid breathing (see p.71).
● Abnormal drowsiness.
● Severe headache.
● Dislike of bright light.
● Refusal to drink for more than 6 hours.

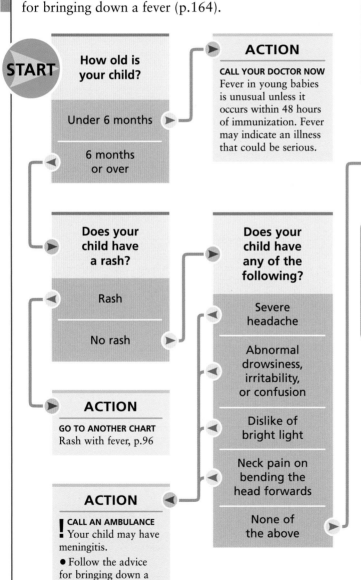

START

How old is your child?

Under 6 months ▶

6 months or over

ACTION

CALL YOUR DOCTOR NOW
Fever in young babies is unusual unless it occurs within 48 hours of immunization. Fever may indicate an illness that could be serious.

Does your child have a rash?

Rash

No rash ▶

ACTION

GO TO ANOTHER CHART
Rash with fever, p.96

ACTION

! **CALL AN AMBULANCE**
Your child may have meningitis.
● Follow the advice for bringing down a fever (p.164).

Does your child have any of the following?

Severe headache

Abnormal drowsiness, irritability, or confusion

Dislike of bright light

Neck pain on bending the head forwards

None of the above

Is your child reluctant to move an arm or leg?

Yes

No ▶

ACTION

CALL YOUR DOCTOR NOW
Your child could have an infection in a bone, such as osteomyelitis, or a joint infection.

ACTION

SEE YOUR DOCTOR WITHIN 24 HOURS
Your child may have acute otitis media (middle-ear infection).
● Give your child liquid paracetamol to relieve pain and reduce fever.

ACTION

! CALL AN AMBULANCE
Your child could have a respiratory infection, such as pneumonia.

● Give your child liquid paracetamol to relieve pain and reduce fever.

Is your child's breathing abnormally noisy or rapid (see p.71)?

Abnormally rapid

Noisy

Neither

ACTION

CALL YOUR DOCTOR NOW
This may be croup, in which a viral infection inflames the airways.

● Sit with your child in a steamy bathroom to ease the breathing.

Does either of the following apply?

Your child has been pulling at one ear

Your child has complained of earache

Neither

Does your child have either of the following?

Cough

Runny nose

Neither

Does your child have a sore throat?

Sore throat

No sore throat

Does your child have either of the following?

Pain on passing urine

Diarrhoea with or without vomiting

Neither

ACTION

SEE YOUR DOCTOR WITHIN 24 HOURS
if you cannot identify a possible cause for your child's fever from this chart.

ACTION

TRY SELF-HELP MEASURES
Your child probably has a viral illness, such as a severe cold or flu.

● Follow the advice for bringing down a fever (p.164).

● Try inhaling steam from a bowl of hot water (p.165).

CONSULT YOUR DOCTOR
if your child's condition worsens, if he or she is no better within 2 days, or if he or she develops other symptoms.

ACTION

TRY SELF-HELP MEASURES
Your child may have a throat infection, such as tonsillitis.

● Follow the advice for bringing down a fever (p.164).

● Follow the advice for soothing a sore throat (p.164).

CONSULT YOUR DOCTOR
if your child is no better in 24 hours or if other symptoms develop.

ACTION

SEE YOUR DOCTOR WITHIN 24 HOURS
Your child may have a urinary tract infection.

● Give plenty of fluids to drink.

ACTION

CALL YOUR DOCTOR NOW
if your child is under 1 year. He or she may have gastroenteritis.

● Give older children plenty of clear fluids to drink.

Excessive sweating

Sweating is one of the body's cooling mechanisms. It is a normal response to heat, exercise, and stress or fear. Some people naturally sweat more than others. Wearing natural fibres, such as cotton, and using an antiperspirant often help to reduce sweating. You should consult your doctor if you sweat excessively and are unsure of the cause.

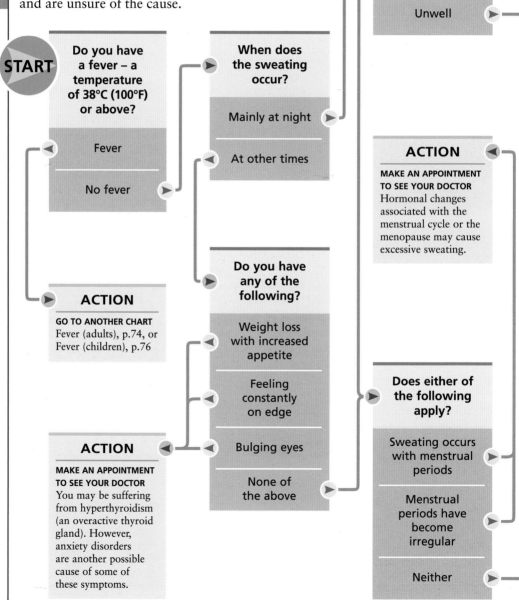

Do you feel otherwise well?

Well

Unwell

START

Do you have a fever – a temperature of 38°C (100°F) or above?

Fever

No fever

When does the sweating occur?

Mainly at night

At other times

ACTION

GO TO ANOTHER CHART
Fever (adults), p.74, or Fever (children), p.76

Do you have any of the following?

Weight loss with increased appetite

Feeling constantly on edge

Bulging eyes

None of the above

ACTION

MAKE AN APPOINTMENT TO SEE YOUR DOCTOR
You may be suffering from hyperthyroidism (an overactive thyroid gland). However, anxiety disorders are another possible cause of some of these symptoms.

ACTION

MAKE AN APPOINTMENT TO SEE YOUR DOCTOR
Hormonal changes associated with the menstrual cycle or the menopause may cause excessive sweating.

Does either of the following apply?

Sweating occurs with menstrual periods

Menstrual periods have become irregular

Neither

ACTION

SEE YOUR DOCTOR WITHIN 24 HOURS
You may have a chronic infection, such as tuberculosis, or a cancer, such as lymphoma (cancer of the lymphatic system).

ACTION

TRY SELF-HELP MEASURES
Being overweight can lead to excessive sweating, particularly after physical exertion.
● Adopt a sensible weight-reducing diet.
● Wash away sweat regularly and wear comfortable loose clothing made from natural fibres.
CONSULT YOUR DOCTOR if your symptoms do not improve.

ACTION

TRY SELF-HELP MEASURES
Excessive sweating of the hands and feet is a common problem.
● Wash away sweat regularly and wear socks made from natural fibres. Try to go barefoot whenever it is possible.
CONSULT YOUR DOCTOR if your symptoms do not improve.

Is your weight within ideal limits?

Overweight

Ideal weight

Underweight

Do you regularly drink more than the recommended limit of alcohol (see box below)?

More than the limit

Within the limit

Is the sweating limited to certain parts of the body?

Mainly hands

Mainly feet

Other parts affected

ACTION

MAKE AN APPOINTMENT TO SEE YOUR DOCTOR
for advice about reducing the amount of alcohol you drink.

ACTION

SEE YOUR DOCTOR WITHIN 24 HOURS
if you cannot identify a possible cause from this chart.

Are you currently taking any medication?

Medication

No medication

ACTION

MAKE AN APPOINTMENT TO SEE YOUR DOCTOR
Your symptoms may be a side effect of the medication.
● Stop taking any over-the-counter medicines but continue to take prescribed medication unless advised to stop by your doctor.

Safe alcohol limits

One unit of alcohol equals half a pint of beer, a small glass of wine or sherry, or a single measure of a spirit.
● The maximum recommended limit for men is 3 units a day.
● The maximum recommended limit for women is 2 units a day.

Lumps and swellings

Enlarged lymph nodes (glands) are often the cause of lumps and swellings under the skin, particularly in the neck, under the arms, or in the groin. These glands usually become swollen due to an infection. The swelling subsides shortly after the infection clears up. If the lumps are painful or if they are persistent but painless, you should consult your doctor.

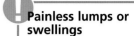

Painless lumps or swellings

Any painless lump or swelling that does not disappear within 2 weeks should be seen by a doctor. Although in most cases the cause is not serious, a painless lump may be a sign of cancer. Early treatment can be life saving.

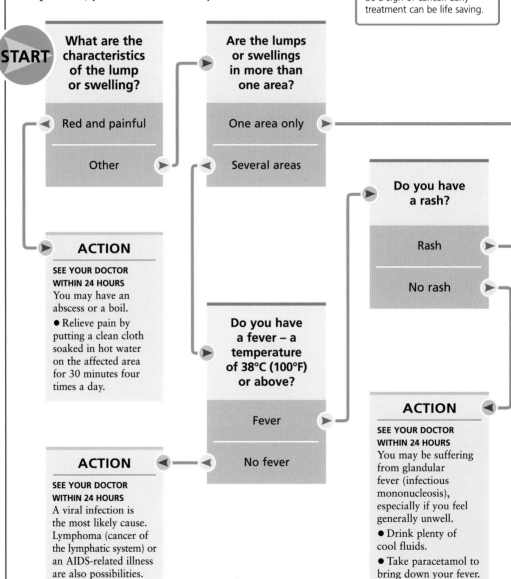

START

What are the characteristics of the lump or swelling?

Red and painful

Other

Are the lumps or swellings in more than one area?

One area only

Several areas

Do you have a rash?

Rash

No rash

ACTION

SEE YOUR DOCTOR WITHIN 24 HOURS
You may have an abscess or a boil.
● Relieve pain by putting a clean cloth soaked in hot water on the affected area for 30 minutes four times a day.

Do you have a fever – a temperature of 38°C (100°F) or above?

Fever

No fever

ACTION

SEE YOUR DOCTOR WITHIN 24 HOURS
You may be suffering from glandular fever (infectious mononucleosis), especially if you feel generally unwell.
● Drink plenty of cool fluids.
● Take paracetamol to bring down your fever.

ACTION

SEE YOUR DOCTOR WITHIN 24 HOURS
A viral infection is the most likely cause. Lymphoma (cancer of the lymphatic system) or an AIDS-related illness are also possibilities.

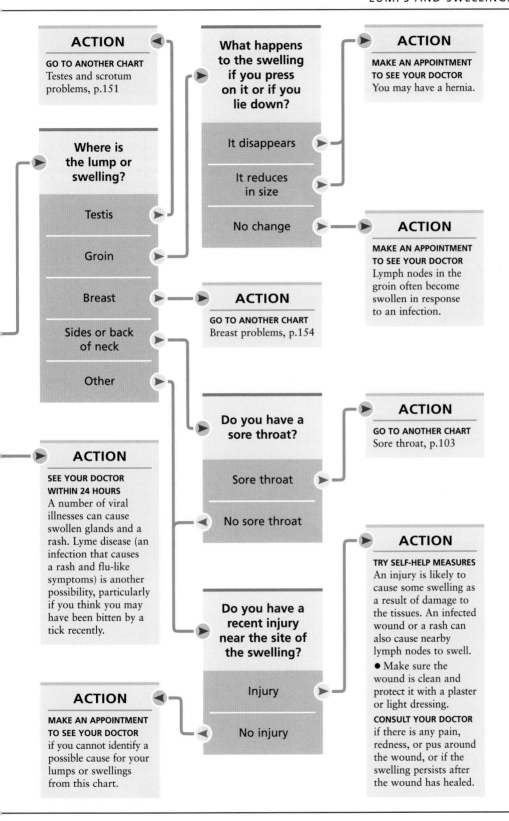

ACTION
GO TO ANOTHER CHART
Testes and scrotum problems, p.151

Where is the lump or swelling?

Testis

Groin

Breast

Sides or back of neck

Other

What happens to the swelling if you press on it or if you lie down?

It disappears

It reduces in size

No change

ACTION
MAKE AN APPOINTMENT TO SEE YOUR DOCTOR
You may have a hernia.

ACTION
MAKE AN APPOINTMENT TO SEE YOUR DOCTOR
Lymph nodes in the groin often become swollen in response to an infection.

ACTION
GO TO ANOTHER CHART
Breast problems, p.154

Do you have a sore throat?

Sore throat

No sore throat

ACTION
GO TO ANOTHER CHART
Sore throat, p.103

ACTION
SEE YOUR DOCTOR WITHIN 24 HOURS
A number of viral illnesses can cause swollen glands and a rash. Lyme disease (an infection that causes a rash and flu-like symptoms) is another possibility, particularly if you think you may have been bitten by a tick recently.

Do you have a recent injury near the site of the swelling?

Injury

No injury

ACTION
MAKE AN APPOINTMENT TO SEE YOUR DOCTOR
if you cannot identify a possible cause for your lumps or swellings from this chart.

ACTION
TRY SELF-HELP MEASURES
An injury is likely to cause some swelling as a result of damage to the tissues. An infected wound or a rash can also cause nearby lymph nodes to swell.
● Make sure the wound is clean and protect it with a plaster or light dressing.
CONSULT YOUR DOCTOR
if there is any pain, redness, or pus around the wound, or if the swelling persists after the wound has healed.

Feeling faint/passing out

A sensation of dizziness or light-headedness may be followed by passing out (loss of consciousness). The cause is usually lack of food or a reduction in blood flow to the brain. A brief episode of feeling faint without other symptoms is not a cause for alarm, but you should consult your doctor if such episodes recur or if you have passed out.

Unconsciousness

If someone remains unconscious for more than a minute or so, whatever the suspected cause, you should get emergency medical help.

- If you need to leave the person to call for help, first lay him or her in the recovery position (pp.14–15).
- Do not move the person if you suspect spinal injury.

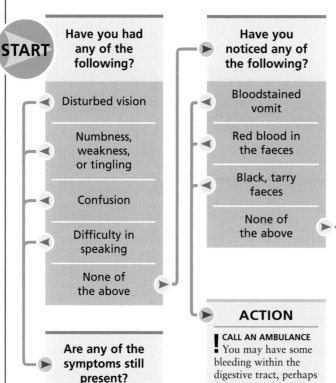

START

Have you had any of the following?

- Disturbed vision
- Numbness, weakness, or tingling
- Confusion
- Difficulty in speaking
- None of the above

Have you noticed any of the following?

- Bloodstained vomit
- Red blood in the faeces
- Black, tarry faeces
- None of the above

Did any of the following occur when you passed out?

- You twitched uncontrollably
- You bit your tongue
- You passed urine
- None of the above

Are any of the symptoms still present?

- Symptoms present
- Symptoms no longer present

ACTION

! **CALL AN AMBULANCE**
You may have some bleeding within the digestive tract, perhaps from a stomach ulcer (an eroded area of the stomach lining) or from an inflammation in the colon.

ACTION

! **CALL AN AMBULANCE**
You may have had a stroke.

ACTION

CALL YOUR DOCTOR NOW
You may have had a mini-stroke.

ACTION

! **CALL AN AMBULANCE**
if this is your first attack. You may have had a seizure, possibly due to epilepsy.

CONSULT YOUR DOCTOR
if you have had previous similar attacks.

ACTION

TRY SELF-HELP MEASURES
Sudden shock can lead to feeling faint or even passing out.
● Rest and ask someone to stay with you until you feel better.
● Follow the first-aid advice for treating fainting (p.53)
CONSULT YOUR DOCTOR
if it happens again.

Does either of the following apply?

You have diabetes

You had not eaten for several hours before passing out

Neither

ACTION

CALL YOUR DOCTOR NOW
Low blood sugar (which may be due to excessive insulin treatment) may be the cause.
● Eat or drink something sugary now.

ACTION

**SEE YOUR DOCTOR
WITHIN 24 HOURS**
You may be anaemic. This can be confirmed by a blood test.

Did you feel faint or pass out immediately after either of the following?

Emotional shock

Getting up suddenly

Neither

Do you have any of the following?

Shortness of breath

Paler skin than normal

Undue tiredness

None of the above

ACTION

**MAKE AN APPOINTMENT
TO SEE YOUR DOCTOR**
Fainting is common in early pregnancy. If you are not sure whether you are pregnant, do a home pregnancy test.

Might you be pregnant?

Possibly pregnant

Not pregnant

ACTION

**SEE YOUR DOCTOR
WITHIN 24 HOURS**
if you passed out, or in the next few days even if you did not pass out. The most likely cause is a temporary drop in blood pressure due to a change in position.

Does either of the following apply?

You have had chest pain or you have a heart condition

You have had palpitations

Neither

ACTION

CALL YOUR DOCTOR NOW
You may have low blood pressure due to an irregular heartbeat or a worsening of an existing heart condition.

ACTION

CALL YOUR DOCTOR NOW
if you passed out and cannot identify a possible cause from this chart.
**SEE YOUR DOCTOR
WITHIN 24 HOURS**
if you cannot identify a possible cause for feeling faint.

Headache

Tension in head and neck muscles and fever are common causes of headache. Too much alcohol, caffeine, or nicotine may also cause a headache. Most headaches do not last for more than a few hours. If your headache lasts for more than 24 hours, is not improved by over-the-counter painkillers, or recurs several times in a week, consult your doctor.

Danger signs

Call an ambulance if a headache is accompanied by any of the following symptoms:
- Drowsiness or confusion.
- Weakness of a limb.
- Blurred vision.
- Dislike of bright light.
- Temporary unconsciousness.

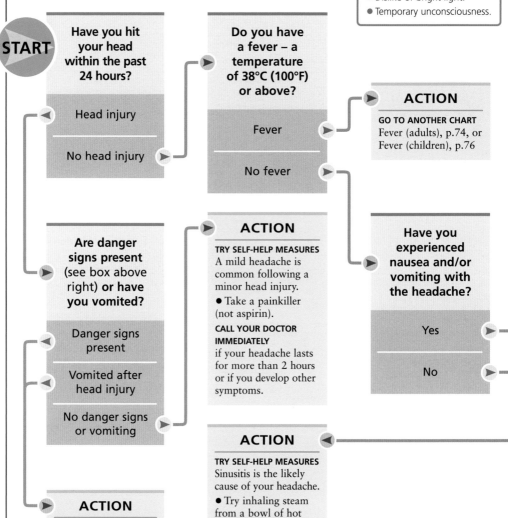

START

Have you hit your head within the past 24 hours?

Head injury

No head injury

Do you have a fever – a temperature of 38°C (100°F) or above?

Fever

No fever

ACTION

GO TO ANOTHER CHART
Fever (adults), p.74, or Fever (children), p.76

Are danger signs present (see box above right) or have you vomited?

Danger signs present

Vomited after head injury

No danger signs or vomiting

ACTION

TRY SELF-HELP MEASURES
A mild headache is common following a minor head injury.
- Take a painkiller (not aspirin).

CALL YOUR DOCTOR IMMEDIATELY
if your headache lasts for more than 2 hours or if you develop other symptoms.

Have you experienced nausea and/or vomiting with the headache?

Yes

No

ACTION

CALL AN AMBULANCE
There may be damage to the tissues that surround the brain.

ACTION

TRY SELF-HELP MEASURES
Sinusitis is the likely cause of your headache.
- Try inhaling steam from a bowl of hot water (p.165).

CONSULT YOUR DOCTOR
if you feel no better within 2 days.

How is your vision?

Blurred vision

Disturbed in other ways

Unchanged

ACTION

CALL YOUR DOCTOR NOW
You have probably a migraine, particularly if any visual problems occurred before the headache. However, the slight chance of a more serious disorder, such as a stroke, needs to be ruled out if this is your first migraine.
● Take a painkiller and sips of water.
● Rest in a darkened, quiet room until the pain lessens.
If you have had any previous attacks, try to identify and avoid potential triggers, such as chocolate.

Does either of the following apply?

The pain is felt chiefly in the areas above and below the eyes

You have recently had a runny or stuffy nose

Neither

ACTION

CALL YOUR DOCTOR NOW
Acute glaucoma (a painful, rapid rise in fluid pressure in the eye) is a possibility, particularly if the pain is around your eye.

Where is the pain?

Over one or both temples

Elsewhere

ACTION

CALL YOUR DOCTOR NOW
You may have temporal arteritis (inflammation of blood vessels in the head), particularly if you are over 50 and are feeling unwell.

ACTION

MAKE AN APPOINTMENT TO SEE YOUR DOCTOR
if you cannot identify a possible cause for your headache from this chart.

ACTION

MAKE AN APPOINTMENT TO SEE YOUR DOCTOR
Your symptoms may be a side effect of the medication.
● Stop taking any over-the-counter medicines but continue to take prescribed medication unless advised to stop by your doctor.

Are you taking any medication?

Medication

No medication

Have you had this type of headache before?

Yes

No

ACTION

MAKE AN APPOINTMENT TO SEE YOUR DOCTOR
A recurrent headache for which there is no obvious cause, such as drinking too much alcohol, should always be investigated fully by your doctor.

Vertigo

The unpleasant sensation that your surroundings are moving around you is known as vertigo. It is often associated with nausea and vomiting. Healthy people may experience vertigo temporarily after a ride at an amusement park or after drinking too much alcohol. You should consult your doctor if you develop vertigo for no obvious reason.

Recurring attacks of vertigo

If you have been experiencing attacks of vertigo, it is very important to avoid certain activities that are potentially hazardous to you and to other people. You should not climb ladders or steep flights of stairs, operate machinery, or drive until the cause of your symptoms has been diagnosed and treated.

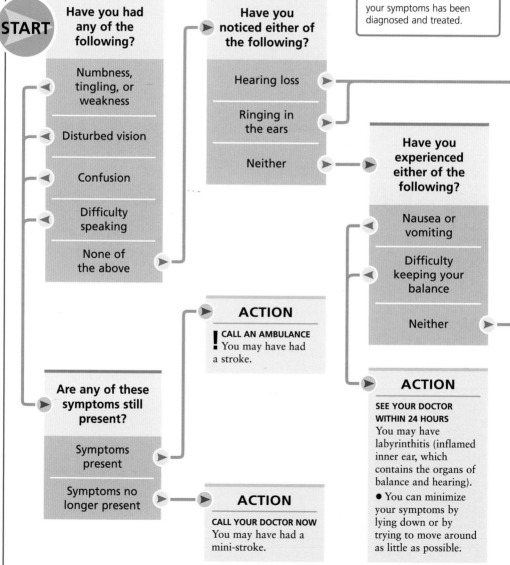

START

Have you had any of the following?

- Numbness, tingling, or weakness
- Disturbed vision
- Confusion
- Difficulty speaking
- None of the above

Have you noticed either of the following?

- Hearing loss
- Ringing in the ears
- Neither

Have you experienced either of the following?

- Nausea or vomiting
- Difficulty keeping your balance
- Neither

Are any of these symptoms still present?

- Symptoms present
- Symptoms no longer present

ACTION

! CALL AN AMBULANCE
You may have had a stroke.

ACTION

CALL YOUR DOCTOR NOW
You may have had a mini-stroke.

ACTION

SEE YOUR DOCTOR WITHIN 24 HOURS
You may have labyrinthitis (inflamed inner ear, which contains the organs of balance and hearing).
● You can minimize your symptoms by lying down or by trying to move around as little as possible.

ACTION

SEE YOUR DOCTOR
WITHIN 24 HOURS
You could be suffering
from Ménière's disease
(a disorder of the inner
ear, which contains
the organs of balance
and hearing).
● Lie still in a darkened
room with your eyes
closed and avoid noise.
Acoustic neuroma
(a noncancerous
tumour of the nerve
that connects the
ear to the brain) is
another, although
less likely, possibility.

ACTION

CALL YOUR DOCTOR NOW
Your symptoms may
be a side effect of your
medication.
● Stop taking any over-
the-counter medicines
but continue to take
prescribed medication
unless advised to stop
by your doctor.

ACTION

TRY SELF-HELP MEASURES
Your symptoms are
most likely to be
caused by drinking
more alcohol than
usual or drinking on
an empty stomach.
● The effects of
alcohol should wear
off within a few hours.
● Meanwhile, drink
plenty of water.
CONSULT YOUR DOCTOR
if the sensation persists
for more than 12 hours.

Are you currently taking any medication?

Medication

No medication

Have you been drinking alcohol?

Yes

No

How old are you?

50 or over

Under 50

ACTION

MAKE AN APPOINTMENT
TO SEE YOUR DOCTOR
Your vertigo may be
caused by osteoarthritis
affecting the bones
and cartilage of the
upper spine (cervical
spondylosis). This can
result in pressure on
blood vessels to the
areas of the brain that
affect balance.
● Try to avoid making
any sudden or extreme
head movements.

Does turning or raising your head bring on vertigo?

Brings on
vertigo

No noticeable
effect

ACTION

SEE YOUR DOCTOR
WITHIN 24 HOURS
if you cannot identify a
possible cause for your
vertigo from this chart.

Numbness and/or tingling

Almost everyone has experienced numbness, the loss of sensation in a part of the body, after sitting or lying in an awkward position for some time. Tingling, a prickly feeling, often occurs as sensation returns to a numb area. You should consult this chart if you experience numbness and/or tingling for which there is no obvious cause.

Danger signs

Call an ambulance if the numbness and/or tingling is accompanied by any of the following symptoms:
- Feeling faint or passing out.
- Disturbed vision.
- Confusion.
- Difficulty speaking.
- Weakness in a limb.

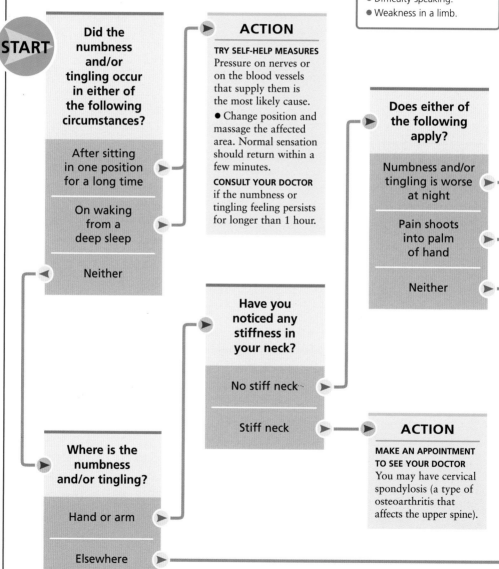

START

Did the numbness and/or tingling occur in either of the following circumstances?

After sitting in one position for a long time

On waking from a deep sleep

Neither

ACTION

TRY SELF-HELP MEASURES Pressure on nerves or on the blood vessels that supply them is the most likely cause.
- Change position and massage the affected area. Normal sensation should return within a few minutes.

CONSULT YOUR DOCTOR if the numbness or tingling feeling persists for longer than 1 hour.

Does either of the following apply?

Numbness and/or tingling is worse at night

Pain shoots into palm of hand

Neither

Have you noticed any stiffness in your neck?

No stiff neck

Stiff neck

ACTION

MAKE AN APPOINTMENT TO SEE YOUR DOCTOR You may have cervical spondylosis (a type of osteoarthritis that affects the upper spine).

Where is the numbness and/or tingling?

Hand or arm

Elsewhere

ACTION

MAKE AN APPOINTMENT TO SEE YOUR DOCTOR
You probably have carpal tunnel syndrome (tingling and pain in the hand and forearm due to a compressed nerve at the wrist).
● Avoid positions that worsen the symptoms.

Have you had any of the following symptoms?

Feeling faint or passing out

Disturbed vision

Confusion

Difficulty speaking

Weakness in a limb

None of the above

ACTION

! CALL AN AMBULANCE
You may have had a stroke.

Are any of these symptoms still present?

Symptoms present

Symptoms no longer present

Are the affected areas on only one side of the body?

One side only

Both sides

Do your fingers become numb and white or blue in either of the following circumstances?

In cold weather

When using vibrating machinery

Neither

ACTION

CALL YOUR DOCTOR NOW
You may have had a mini-stroke.

ACTION

MAKE AN APPOINTMENT TO SEE YOUR DOCTOR
This type of numbness is most likely to be caused by hand–arm syndrome, which is associated with the long-term use of vibrating machinery.
● Avoid using vibrating machinery.
● Keep warm.
● If you smoke, stop.

ACTION

MAKE AN APPOINTMENT TO SEE YOUR DOCTOR
if you cannot identify a possible cause for your numbness and/or tingling from this chart.

ACTION

MAKE AN APPOINTMENT TO SEE YOUR DOCTOR
You may be suffering from Raynaud's phenomenon, in which there is intermittent narrowing of blood vessels in the hands or, rarely, the feet.
● Keep your hands and/or feet warm.
● If you smoke, stop.

Facial pain

Pain in the face may be sharp and stabbing or dull and throbbing, and is most often caused by an inflammation of structures in the face, such as the sinuses or teeth. Facial pain is usually short-lived, but some types, such as neuralgia, may persist. Consult your doctor if the pain is persistent, unexplained, or is not relieved by painkillers.

START

Where is the pain?

- Over one or both temples
- In or around the eye
- Elsewhere

Do any of the following apply?

- Your scalp is sensitive to touch
- You have been feeling unwell
- Pain comes on when chewing
- None of the above

ACTION

GO TO ANOTHER CHART
Painful or irritated eye, p.98

ACTION

CALL YOUR DOCTOR NOW
You may have temporal arteritis (inflammation of blood vessels around the head), especially if you are over 50.

ACTION

MAKE AN APPOINTMENT TO SEE YOUR DOCTOR
You may have trigeminal neuralgia (severe pain due to an irritated nerve).
● Try to avoid triggers if possible.

ACTION

MAKE AN APPOINTMENT TO SEE YOUR DOCTOR OR DENTIST
You may have a disorder in the joint between the jaw and the skull.
● Take paracetamol to relieve the pain.
● Hold a wrapped hot-water bottle against the affected area.

Which of the following describes your pain?

- Stabbing pain when touching the face or chewing
- Aching pain on chewing and/or yawning
- Dull aching around one or both cheekbones
- None of the above

ACTION

TRY SELF-HELP MEASURES
You probably have sinusitis, especially if you have recently had a cold and both sides of your face are affected. If only one side is affected, a dental problem, such as an abscess, is more likely.
● Take a painkiller such as paracetamol.
● Try inhaling steam from a bowl of hot water (p.165) if you think you have sinusitis.
CONSULT YOUR DOCTOR OR DENTIST
if you do not feel better within 2 days.

ACTION

MAKE AN APPOINTMENT TO SEE YOUR DOCTOR
if you cannot identify a possible cause for your facial pain from this chart.

Difficulty speaking

Slurred or unclear speech and the inability to find or use words are symptoms that may have an obvious cause, such as drinking too much alcohol. Developing a difficulty with speaking could also signal a more serious condition affecting the brain's speech centres. If your speech suddenly deteriorates, consult your doctor urgently.

ACTION

! **CALL AN AMBULANCE**
You may have had a stroke.

START

Have you had any of the following?

Are any symptoms still present?

ACTION

CALL YOUR DOCTOR NOW
You may have had a mini-stroke.

Disturbed vision

Numbness, tingling, or weakness

Symptoms present

Symptoms no longer present

ACTION

SEE YOUR DOCTOR WITHIN 24 HOURS
Your symptoms may be a side effect of medication or drugs.
● Stop taking any over-the-counter medicines but continue to take prescribed medication unless advised to stop by your doctor.

Feeling faint or passing out

Confusion

Inability to move the muscles on one side of the face

ACTION

CALL YOUR DOCTOR NOW
You may have a type of facial palsy, such as Bell's palsy, due to damaged facial nerves.
● Take care of your eye as it may not close fully.

None of the above

Do any of these apply?

ACTION

MAKE AN APPOINTMENT TO SEE YOUR DOCTOR for advice on reducing your alcohol intake.

ACTION

MAKE AN APPOINTMENT TO SEE YOUR DOCTOR
You may have glossitis (inflamed tongue).
● Rinse your mouth regularly with a salt solution or an antiseptic or pain-relieving mouthwash.
● Avoid acidic and spicy foods.
● If you smoke, stop.

You have been taking drugs or medication

You have been drinking alcohol

You have a sore mouth or tongue

None of the above

ACTION

SEE YOUR DOCTOR WITHIN 24 HOURS
if you cannot identify a possible cause for your speech difficulty from this chart.

Forgetfulness or confusion

Most people are forgetful sometimes, especially if they are very busy. Absent-mindedness is also a natural part of the aging process. Confusion is the inability to think clearly and may include forgetfulness. You should consult your doctor if episodes of forgetfulness and/or confusion occur frequently or are severe enough to disrupt your life.

Sudden onset of confusion

Phone a doctor immediately if a person suddenly becomes very confused or disoriented about time or place or seems to be seeing or hearing things that are not there.

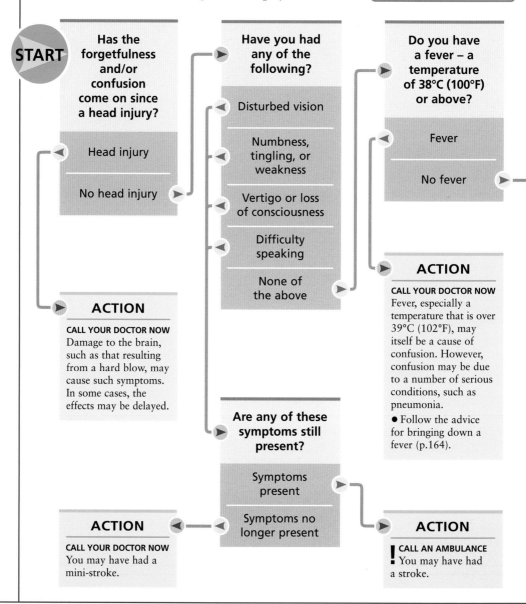

START

Has the forgetfulness and/or confusion come on since a head injury?

Head injury

No head injury

Have you had any of the following?

Disturbed vision

Numbness, tingling, or weakness

Vertigo or loss of consciousness

Difficulty speaking

None of the above

Do you have a fever – a temperature of 38°C (100°F) or above?

Fever

No fever

ACTION

CALL YOUR DOCTOR NOW
Damage to the brain, such as that resulting from a hard blow, may cause such symptoms. In some cases, the effects may be delayed.

ACTION

CALL YOUR DOCTOR NOW
Fever, especially a temperature that is over 39°C (102°F), may itself be a cause of confusion. However, confusion may be due to a number of serious conditions, such as pneumonia.
● Follow the advice for bringing down a fever (p.164).

Are any of these symptoms still present?

Symptoms present

Symptoms no longer present

ACTION

CALL YOUR DOCTOR NOW
You may have had a mini-stroke.

ACTION

! CALL AN AMBULANCE
You may have had a stroke.

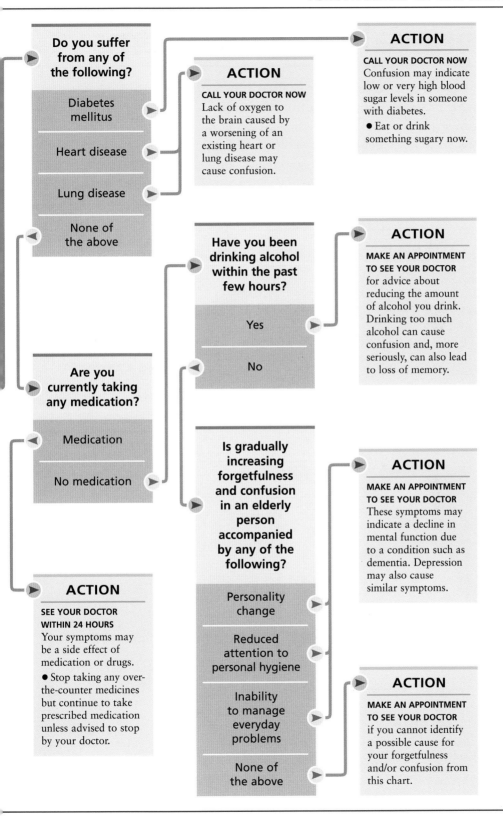

Do you suffer from any of the following?

Diabetes mellitus

Heart disease

Lung disease

None of the above

ACTION

CALL YOUR DOCTOR NOW
Lack of oxygen to the brain caused by a worsening of an existing heart or lung disease may cause confusion.

ACTION

CALL YOUR DOCTOR NOW
Confusion may indicate low or very high blood sugar levels in someone with diabetes.
● Eat or drink something sugary now.

Are you currently taking any medication?

Medication

No medication

Have you been drinking alcohol within the past few hours?

Yes

No

ACTION

MAKE AN APPOINTMENT TO SEE YOUR DOCTOR
for advice about reducing the amount of alcohol you drink. Drinking too much alcohol can cause confusion and, more seriously, can also lead to loss of memory.

ACTION

SEE YOUR DOCTOR WITHIN 24 HOURS
Your symptoms may be a side effect of medication or drugs.
● Stop taking any over-the-counter medicines but continue to take prescribed medication unless advised to stop by your doctor.

Is gradually increasing forgetfulness and confusion in an elderly person accompanied by any of the following?

Personality change

Reduced attention to personal hygiene

Inability to manage everyday problems

None of the above

ACTION

MAKE AN APPOINTMENT TO SEE YOUR DOCTOR
These symptoms may indicate a decline in mental function due to a condition such as dementia. Depression may also cause similar symptoms.

ACTION

MAKE AN APPOINTMENT TO SEE YOUR DOCTOR
if you cannot identify a possible cause for your forgetfulness and/or confusion from this chart.

General skin problems

Skin problems are often caused by localized infection, allergy, or irritation. They are not usually serious, although widespread skin problems may be distressing. You should consult your doctor if: a skin problem lasts more than a month or causes severe discomfort; a new lump appears, especially if it is dark-coloured; or a sore fails to heal.

START

What type of skin problem do you have?

Rash

Other skin problem

Do you have a fever – a temperature of 38°C (100°F) or above?

Fever

No fever

ACTION

GO TO ANOTHER CHART
Rash with fever, p.96

Is the affected skin itchy?

Itchy

Not itchy

What does the area look like?

Painful, blistery rash in one area

Reddened patches covered with silvery scales

Blistery, oozing rash on or around the lips

A painful red lump with a yellow centre

None of the above

ACTION

SEE YOUR DOCTOR WITHIN 24 HOURS
You may have cellulitis (infection of the skin and underlying tissue).

Have you noticed any of the following?

Red, tender, and hot area of skin

New mole or a change in an existing mole

An open sore that has not healed after 3 weeks

None of the above

ACTION

MAKE AN APPOINTMENT TO SEE YOUR DOCTOR
You may possibly have skin cancer.

ACTION

TRY SELF-HELP MEASURES
This may be a boil.
• Apply a hot cloth for 30 mins, 4 times a day.
CONSULT YOUR DOCTOR if the condition has not improved in 24 hours.

What does the affected skin look like?

Areas of inflamed skin with a scaly surface

One or more red bumps with a central dark spot

Intermittent red raised areas (weals)

None of the above

What do the edges of the rash look like?

Merge into surrounding skin

Clearly defined margins

ACTION

MAKE AN APPOINTMENT TO SEE YOUR DOCTOR
You may have a fungal infection like ringworm.

ACTION

TRY SELF-HELP MEASURES
You may have been bitten by an insect.
• Try using an antihistamine cream.

Does either of the following apply?

You have a rash that spreads out from a central red spot

You have been bitten by a tick

Neither

ACTION

SEE YOUR DOCTOR WITHIN 24 HOURS
You may have impetigo.
• Do not touch blisters.
If you have had the same problem before, it could be a cold sore.
• Use an over-the-counter antiviral cream.

ACTION

TRY SELF-HELP MEASURES
You may have a form of eczema.
• Follow the advice for relieving itchiness (p.165).
CONSULT YOUR DOCTOR
if your rash does not improve within 1 week or if any other symptoms develop.

ACTION

TRY SELF-HELP MEASURES
You may have urticaria.
• Soothe the irritation with cold compresses or calamine lotion.
• Try over-the-counter antihistamine tablets.
CALL YOUR DOCTOR NOW
if you are experiencing breathing difficulties.

ACTION

SEE YOUR DOCTOR WITHIN 24 HOURS
You may have shingles.
• Soothe the irritation with cold compresses or calamine lotion.
• Take a painkiller such as paracetamol.

ACTION

MAKE AN APPOINTMENT TO SEE YOUR DOCTOR
You may have psoriasis.

ACTION

SEE YOUR DOCTOR WITHIN 24 HOURS
You may have Lyme disease, which is carried by ticks.

ACTION

CALL YOUR DOCTOR NOW
Your symptoms may be a side effect of the drug.
• Stop taking any over-the-counter medicines but continue to take prescribed medication unless advised to stop by your doctor.

Are you currently taking any medication?

Medication

No medication

ACTION

MAKE AN APPOINTMENT TO SEE YOUR DOCTOR
if you cannot identify a possible cause for your skin problem from this chart.

Rash with fever

◀ **For rash without fever, see p.94**

If you or your child has a temperature of 38°C (100°F) or above, you should check whether a rash is also present. A rash with fever is usually caused by a viral infection, most of which are not serious. However, a rash may alert you to the possibility of potentially life-threatening meningitis.

Danger signs

Call an ambulance if a rash and fever are accompanied by any of the following:
- Abnormal drowsiness.
- Seizures.
- Temperature of 39°C (102°F) or above.
- Abnormally rapid breathing (see advice on checking your child's breathing rate, p.71).
- Noisy or difficult breathing.
- Severe headache.

START

What are the features of the rash?

- Widespread itchy, blistery rash
- Rash that spreads from a central red spot
- Flat, dark red spots that do not fade when pressed
- Dull red spots or blotches that fade when pressed
- Bright red rash, particularly on the cheeks
- Pale pink, widespread rash
- None of the above

ACTION

SEE YOUR DOCTOR WITHIN 24 HOURS

You may have chickenpox, which may need treatment with an antiviral drug.
- Follow the advice for bringing down a fever (p.164).
- Apply calamine lotion to relieve the itchiness of the rash.

ACTION

SEE YOUR DOCTOR WITHIN 24 HOURS

You may have Lyme disease (an infection transmitted by ticks that causes a rash and flu-like symptoms).
- Follow the advice for bringing down a fever (p.164).

ACTION

SEE YOUR DOCTOR WITHIN 24 HOURS

Fifth disease (or slapped cheek disease) due to a parvovirus infection may be the cause in a child.
- Follow the advice for bringing down a fever (p.164).

ACTION

SEE YOUR DOCTOR WITHIN 24 HOURS

You may have rubella (German measles). Roseola infantum (a viral infection that causes high fever followed by a rash of tiny pink spots) is another possibility, particularly in children under 4 years old.
- Follow the advice for bringing down a fever (p.164).
- Warn any contact you think could be pregnant.

ACTION

SEE YOUR DOCTOR WITHIN 24 HOURS if you cannot identify a possible cause for your rash and fever from this chart.

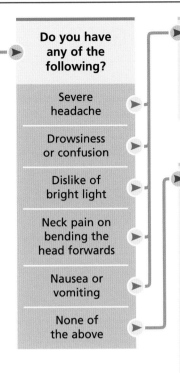

Do you have any of the following?

Severe headache

Drowsiness or confusion

Dislike of bright light

Neck pain on bending the head forwards

Nausea or vomiting

None of the above

ACTION

! CALL AN AMBULANCE
You may have meningitis (inflamed membranes around the brain).

ACTION

CALL YOUR DOCTOR NOW
This type of rash may be due to a severe allergic reaction to a drug such as penicillin. It could also be the result of a blood disorder that causes bleeding into the skin.
● Stop taking any over-the-counter medicines but continue to take prescribed medication unless advised to stop by your doctor.

Checking a red rash
If you develop a dark red rash, check if it fades on pressure by pressing the side of a drinking glass on to it. If the rash is visible through the glass, it may be a form of purpura, a rash caused by bleeding from tiny blood vessels in the skin either because blood vessels are damaged or because of an abnormality in the blood. Purpura can be caused by one of several serious disorders, including meningitis, and needs prompt medical attention. Call an ambulance if you have a high fever, severe headache, or any of the other danger signs listed opposite.

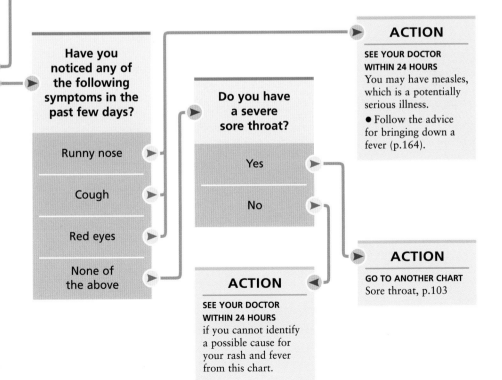

Have you noticed any of the following symptoms in the past few days?

Runny nose

Cough

Red eyes

None of the above

Do you have a severe sore throat?

Yes

No

ACTION

SEE YOUR DOCTOR WITHIN 24 HOURS
You may have measles, which is a potentially serious illness.
● Follow the advice for bringing down a fever (p.164).

ACTION

GO TO ANOTHER CHART
Sore throat, p.103

ACTION

SEE YOUR DOCTOR WITHIN 24 HOURS
if you cannot identify a possible cause for your rash and fever from this chart.

Painful or irritated eye

Injury, infection, and allergy are the most common causes of discomfort or irritation of the eye and eyelids. A painless red area in the white of the eye is likely to be a burst blood vessel and should clear up without treatment. However, you should see your doctor if your eyes are sore. Consult your doctor immediately if your vision deteriorates.

Contact lens wearers

If you wear contact lenses and experience any kind of eye pain or irritation:
- Remove your lenses without delay.
- Do not use them again until the problem has been identified and treated. If the pain is caused by grit under the lens, there is a risk that the cornea will be scratched.
- Make an appointment to see your optician.

START

Does either of the following apply?

You have something in your eye

You have injured your eye

Neither

ACTION

TRY SELF-HELP MEASURES
A foreign object in your eye is likely to cause pain and redness.
- Follow the first-aid advice for dealing with a foreign object in the eye (p.36).

SEEK EMERGENCY HELP IN HOSPITAL
if a foreign object is embedded in the eye.

What is the main symptom?

Pain in and around the eye

Itching or irritation of the eyelid

Tender red lump on the eyelid

The eye feels gritty

None of the above

Has your vision deteriorated since the injury?

Yes

No

ACTION

TRY SELF-HELP MEASURES
You may have a stye (infected hair follicle) or a chalazion (infected gland in the eyelid).
- Hold a clean, warm, damp cloth on the eyelid for 20 minutes several times a day.

CONSULT YOUR DOCTOR
if your eye does not improve within 3 days.

ACTION

SEE YOUR DOCTOR WITHIN 24 HOURS
Your pain may be due to a minor eye injury.
- Follow the first-aid advice for dealing with eye wounds (p.35).

ACTION

CALL AN AMBULANCE
A serious eye injury is possible. Expert help may be needed to prevent permanent damage to the eye.

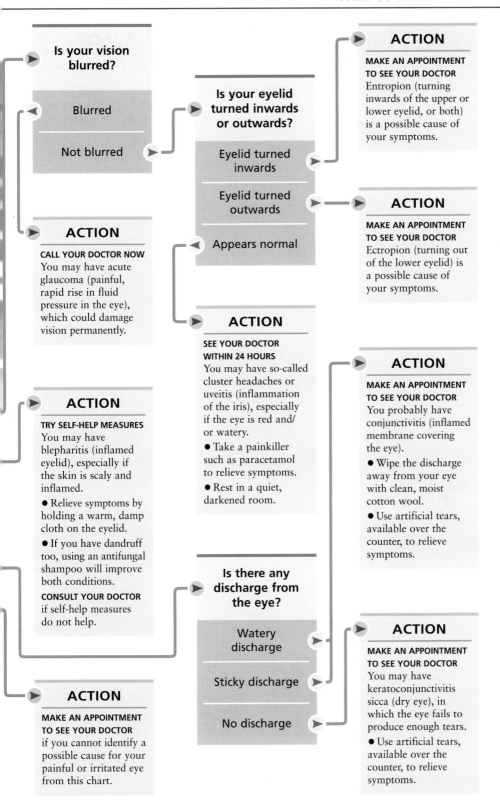

Is your vision blurred?

Blurred

Not blurred

Is your eyelid turned inwards or outwards?

Eyelid turned inwards

Eyelid turned outwards

Appears normal

ACTION

MAKE AN APPOINTMENT TO SEE YOUR DOCTOR
Entropion (turning inwards of the upper or lower eyelid, or both) is a possible cause of your symptoms.

ACTION

MAKE AN APPOINTMENT TO SEE YOUR DOCTOR
Ectropion (turning out of the lower eyelid) is a possible cause of your symptoms.

ACTION

CALL YOUR DOCTOR NOW
You may have acute glaucoma (painful, rapid rise in fluid pressure in the eye), which could damage vision permanently.

ACTION

SEE YOUR DOCTOR WITHIN 24 HOURS
You may have so-called cluster headaches or uveitis (inflammation of the iris), especially if the eye is red and/or watery.
● Take a painkiller such as paracetamol to relieve symptoms.
● Rest in a quiet, darkened room.

ACTION

MAKE AN APPOINTMENT TO SEE YOUR DOCTOR
You probably have conjunctivitis (inflamed membrane covering the eye).
● Wipe the discharge away from your eye with clean, moist cotton wool.
● Use artificial tears, available over the counter, to relieve symptoms.

ACTION

TRY SELF-HELP MEASURES
You may have blepharitis (inflamed eyelid), especially if the skin is scaly and inflamed.
● Relieve symptoms by holding a warm, damp cloth on the eyelid.
● If you have dandruff too, using an antifungal shampoo will improve both conditions.
CONSULT YOUR DOCTOR if self-help measures do not help.

Is there any discharge from the eye?

Watery discharge

Sticky discharge

No discharge

ACTION

MAKE AN APPOINTMENT TO SEE YOUR DOCTOR
if you cannot identify a possible cause for your painful or irritated eye from this chart.

ACTION

MAKE AN APPOINTMENT TO SEE YOUR DOCTOR
You may have keratoconjunctivitis sicca (dry eye), in which the eye fails to produce enough tears.
● Use artificial tears, available over the counter, to relieve symptoms.

Disturbed/impaired vision

Visual disturbances might include blurred vision or seeing double. You may also see flashing lights or floating spots. These disturbances may be caused by a problem in one or both eyes or by damage to the areas in the brain that process visual information. If your vision deteriorates suddenly, you should consult your doctor immediately.

START

Do you have pain in the affected eye?

Pain

No pain

ACTION

GO TO ANOTHER CHART
Painful or irritated eye, p.98

How long has your vision been disturbed or impaired?

Less than 24 hours

24 hours or longer

Do you have diabetes?

Yes

No

ACTION

SEE YOUR DOCTOR
WITHIN 24 HOURS
Damage to blood vessels in the retina due to diabetes or high blood sugar levels can lead to blurred vision.

How old are you?

50 or over

Under 50

ACTION

! CALL AN AMBULANCE
You may have damaged the part of the brain that is responsible for vision.

Have you injured your head in the past 48 hours?

Recent head injury

No head injury

ACTION

MAKE AN APPOINTMENT TO SEE YOUR DOCTOR
A cataract (clouding of the lens of the eye) can cause blurred vision in older people.

What kind of visual disturbance or impairment have you been experiencing?

Blurred vision

Increasing difficulty in focusing on nearby objects

Other disturbance

What is the nature of your disturbed or impaired vision?

- Sudden loss of all or part of the vision in one or both eyes
- Blurred vision
- Seeing flashing lights or floating spots
- Double vision
- None of the above

ACTION

! CALL AN AMBULANCE
You may have blockage of a blood vessel that supplies the brain or eye. Another possibility is a detached retina, which needs prompt treatment.

ACTION

CALL YOUR DOCTOR NOW
You may have a migraine. However, the possibility of another disorder needs to be ruled out.
- Rest in a darkened quiet room until symptoms improve.
- If you also have a headache, take a painkiller such as paracetamol.

CONSULT YOUR DOCTOR
if you have had previous migraines.
- Avoid red wine, chocolate, and mature cheese – all possible migraine triggers.

ACTION

! CALL AN AMBULANCE
This may be due to bleeding in the brain, such as with a stroke or subarachnoid haemorrhage (ruptured artery near the brain). Another possibility is a weakness or paralysis of the muscles that control the movement of the eyes, causing double vision.

ACTION

SEE YOUR DOCTOR WITHIN 24 HOURS
Your symptoms may be a side effect of the medication.
- Stop taking any over-the-counter medicines but continue to take prescribed medication unless advised to stop by your doctor.

ACTION

CALL YOUR DOCTOR NOW
if you cannot identify a possible cause for your disturbed or impaired vision from this chart.

ACTION

MAKE AN APPOINTMENT TO SEE YOUR OPTICIAN
You may be developing presbyopia (gradual loss of the eyes' ability to focus on near objects) as part of the normal aging process.

Are you currently taking any medication?

- Medication
- No medication

ACTION

SEE YOUR DOCTOR WITHIN 24 HOURS
if you cannot identify a possible cause for your disturbed or impaired vision from this chart.

Earache

Pain in one or both ears is a distressing symptom, especially for children. Earache is usually caused by an infection in the outer or middle ear. Mild discomfort, however, may be due to wax blockage. Consult your doctor if you suffer from earache, particularly if it is persistent. A severe or recurrent middle-ear infection may damage hearing.

START

Does pulling the ear lobe make the pain worse?

Increases pain

Pain is no worse

ACTION

MAKE AN APPOINTMENT TO SEE YOUR DOCTOR
Your earache is probably due to otitis externa (infection of the outer ear) or a boil in the ear canal.
● Take a painkiller such as paracetamol.

ACTION

SEE YOUR DOCTOR WITHIN 24 HOURS
You may have otitis media (middle-ear infection) with a perforated eardrum; otitis externa (outer-ear infection) is another possibility.
● Take a painkiller such as paracetamol.

ACTION

MAKE AN APPOINTMENT TO SEE YOUR DOCTOR
if the discomfort persists for longer than 24 hours. Barotrauma (ear damage or pain caused by pressure changes) may be the cause of your pain.

Is there a discharge from the affected ear?

Discharge

No discharge

ACTION

TRY SELF-HELP MEASURES
A cold may often be accompanied by mild earache. Persistent or severe earache is likely to be due to otitis media (middle-ear infection).
● Take a decongestant to relieve stuffiness and a painkiller, such as paracetamol, to relieve discomfort.
CONSULT YOUR DOCTOR
if the pain is severe or if it persists for longer than 2 days.

Did the pain start during or immediately after an aeroplane flight?

During or immediately after

Unrelated to air travel

Do you have a runny or stuffy nose?

Yes

No

ACTION

SEE YOUR DOCTOR WITHIN 24 HOURS
if you cannot identify a possible cause for your earache from this chart.

Sore throat

A raw or rough feeling in the throat is a symptom that most people have from time to time. A sore throat is often the first sign of a common cold and is also a feature of other viral infections. You can treat a sore throat yourself at home unless you also have other, more serious symptoms. However, if your sore throat persists or is severe, consult your doctor.

START

Do you have a fever – a temperature of 38°C (100°F) or above?

Fever

No fever

Do you have swelling in your groin and/or armpits ?

Yes

No

ACTION

MAKE AN APPOINTMENT TO SEE YOUR DOCTOR
You may be suffering from glandular fever (infectious mononucleosis).

Do you have any of these?

Generalized aches and pains

Runny nose

Headache

Cough

None of the above

ACTION

MAKE AN APPOINTMENT TO SEE YOUR DOCTOR
You may have either tonsillitis or pharyngitis (inflamed throat).
● Follow the advice for soothing a sore throat (p.164).

ACTION

TRY SELF-HELP MEASURES
Activities such as these are likely to result in pharyngitis (inflamed throat) or tonsillitis, or both.
● Follow the advice for soothing a sore throat (p.164).
CONSULT YOUR DOCTOR
if your symptoms worsen, change, or are no better in 2 days.

ACTION

TRY SELF-HELP MEASURES
You probably have a severe cold or flu.
● Follow the advice for bringing down a fever (p.164).
CONSULT YOUR DOCTOR
if your symptoms worsen, change, or are no better after 2 days.

Before the onset of your sore throat, had you been doing any of these?

Smoking heavily or breathing smoke

Shouting or singing loudly

None of the above

ACTION

TRY SELF-HELP MEASURES
You may have a cold.
● Follow the advice for soothing a sore throat (p.164).
CONSULT YOUR DOCTOR
if you are no better within 2 days.

Hoarseness or loss of voice

The sudden onset of hoarseness or huskiness of the voice is a common symptom of upper respiratory tract infections that involve the larynx or vocal cords. Such infections are almost always caused by viruses. Hoarseness and loss of voice that develop gradually are most commonly caused by overuse of the voice, smoking, or, rarely, cancer of the larynx.

Persistent change in the voice

It is important to seek medical advice if you develop hoarseness or any other voice change that lasts for more than 2 weeks, since the slight possibility of cancer of the larynx needs to be ruled out.

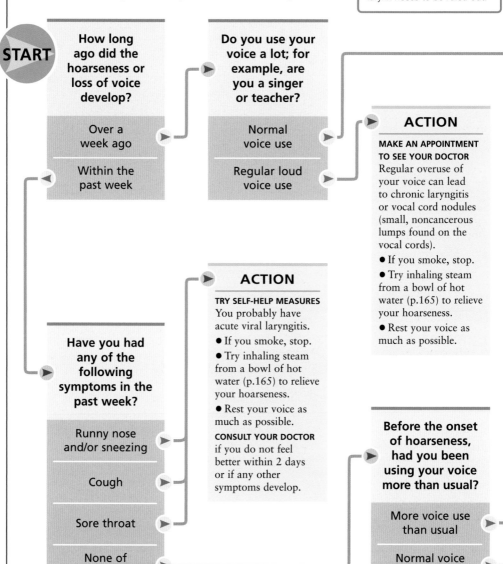

START

How long ago did the hoarseness or loss of voice develop?

- Over a week ago
- Within the past week

Do you use your voice a lot; for example, are you a singer or teacher?

- Normal voice use
- Regular loud voice use

ACTION

MAKE AN APPOINTMENT TO SEE YOUR DOCTOR Regular overuse of your voice can lead to chronic laryngitis or vocal cord nodules (small, noncancerous lumps found on the vocal cords).

- If you smoke, stop.
- Try inhaling steam from a bowl of hot water (p.165) to relieve your hoarseness.
- Rest your voice as much as possible.

Have you had any of the following symptoms in the past week?

- Runny nose and/or sneezing
- Cough
- Sore throat
- None of the above

ACTION

TRY SELF-HELP MEASURES You probably have acute viral laryngitis.

- If you smoke, stop.
- Try inhaling steam from a bowl of hot water (p.165) to relieve your hoarseness.
- Rest your voice as much as possible.

CONSULT YOUR DOCTOR if you do not feel better within 2 days or if any other symptoms develop.

Before the onset of hoarseness, had you been using your voice more than usual?

- More voice use than usual
- Normal voice use

Do you smoke, or have you smoked in the past?

Yes

No

ACTION

MAKE AN APPOINTMENT TO SEE YOUR DOCTOR
Heavy smoking over a long period of time can result in laryngitis.
● If you smoke, stop.
● Rest your voice as much as possible.
Another possibility is cancer of the larynx, which is more common in regular smokers.

ACTION

MAKE AN APPOINTMENT TO SEE YOUR DOCTOR
Hypothyroidism (underactivity of the thyroid gland) can cause a husky voice.

ACTION

TRY SELF-HELP MEASURES
Excessive use of the voice can inflame the vocal cords.
● If you smoke, stop.
● Try inhaling steam from a bowl of hot water (p.165) to relieve your hoarseness.
● Rest your voice as much as possible.
CONSULT YOUR DOCTOR
if your voice is no better within 2 days or if any other symptoms develop.

ACTION

CALL YOUR DOCTOR NOW
Breathing in dust, fumes, or smoke can inflame the airways.

Do you have any of the following?

Tiredness

Increased skin dryness or roughness

Feeling the cold more than you used to

Unexplained weight gain

Generalized hair thinning

None of the above

ACTION

TRY SELF-HELP MEASURES
Being in a smoky atmosphere can inflame the vocal cords.
● If you smoke, stop.
● Try inhaling steam from a bowl of hot water (p.165) to relieve your hoarseness.
● Rest your voice as much as possible.
CONSULT YOUR DOCTOR
if your voice is no better within 2 days or if any other symptoms develop.

Did either of the following apply before the onset of hoarseness?

You had inhaled dust, chemical fumes, or smoke from a fire

You had spent time in a smoky atmosphere

Neither

ACTION

MAKE AN APPOINTMENT TO SEE YOUR DOCTOR
if you cannot identify a possible cause for your hoarseness or loss of voice from this chart.

Coughing (adults)

For children under 12, see p.108 ▶
Coughing is the body's defence mechanism for clearing the airways of inhaled particles or secretions. Persistent coughing may be due to infection or inflammation in the lungs or to the effects of irritants such as tobacco smoke. Persistent coughing should be investigated by your doctor.

❗ Coughing up blood
If you cough up sputum that contains streaks of blood on one occasion only, the most likely cause is a small tear in the lining of the windpipe; if you feel well, you need not be concerned. However, if you have more than one such episode, there may be a more serious cause; you should see a doctor without delay.

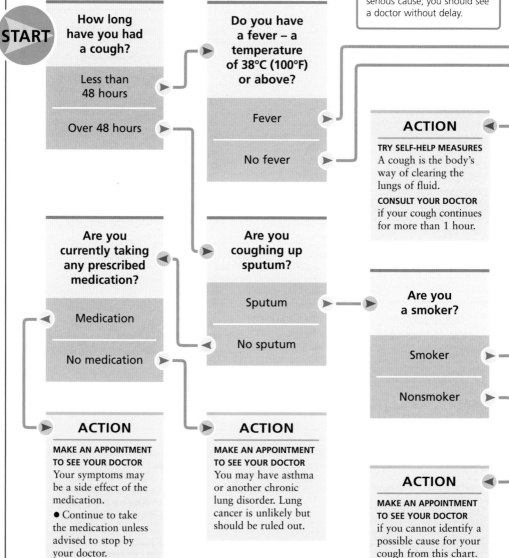

START

How long have you had a cough?

Less than 48 hours ▶

Over 48 hours ▶

Do you have a fever – a temperature of 38°C (100°F) or above?

Fever ▶

No fever ▶

ACTION

TRY SELF-HELP MEASURES A cough is the body's way of clearing the lungs of fluid.

CONSULT YOUR DOCTOR if your cough continues for more than 1 hour.

Are you currently taking any prescribed medication?

Medication ◀

No medication ▶

Are you coughing up sputum?

Sputum ▶

No sputum ◀

Are you a smoker?

Smoker ▶

Nonsmoker ▶

ACTION

MAKE AN APPOINTMENT TO SEE YOUR DOCTOR Your symptoms may be a side effect of the medication.

● Continue to take the medication unless advised to stop by your doctor.

ACTION

MAKE AN APPOINTMENT TO SEE YOUR DOCTOR You may have asthma or another chronic lung disorder. Lung cancer is unlikely but should be ruled out.

ACTION

MAKE AN APPOINTMENT TO SEE YOUR DOCTOR if you cannot identify a possible cause for your cough from this chart.

Do you have either of the following?

Pain on breathing

Shortness of breath

Neither

ACTION

CALL YOUR DOCTOR NOW
You may have pneumonia.

● Take paracetamol to help reduce your fever and pain.

Have you coughed up sputum?

Sputum

No sputum

ACTION

TRY SELF-HELP MEASURES
You may have acute bronchitis.

● Take paracetamol to reduce your fever and chest pain.

● Drink plenty of fluids.

● If you smoke, stop.

CONSULT YOUR DOCTOR
if your symptoms worsen or if you are no better within 2 days.

Have you inhaled any of these in the last few hours?

Particle of food

Tobacco smoke

Dust, fumes, or smoke from a fire

None of the above

ACTION

CALL YOUR DOCTOR NOW
Inflammation of the airways can result from breathing in any of these substances.

ACTION

TRY SELF-HELP MEASURES
You may have a viral illness such as a severe cold or flu.

● Follow the advice for bringing down a fever (p.164).

● Try inhaling steam from a bowl of hot water (p.165) to relieve your symptoms.

MAKE AN APPOINTMENT TO SEE YOUR DOCTOR
if you are no better in 2 days or if other symptoms develop.

Do you have either of the following?

Runny nose

Sore throat

Neither

ACTION

TRY SELF-HELP MEASURES
Smoke can irritate the lungs.

● Move into a well-ventilated area.

ACTION

TRY SELF-HELP MEASURES
You probably have a viral infection, such as a cold.

● Try inhaling steam from a bowl of hot water (p.165) to relieve your symptoms.

MAKE AN APPOINTMENT TO SEE YOUR DOCTOR
if you are no better in 2 days or if other symptoms develop.

ACTION

MAKE AN APPOINTMENT TO SEE YOUR DOCTOR
You may have chronic lung damage from smoking or possibly lung cancer.

● If you smoke, give up immediately.

ACTION

MAKE AN APPOINTMENT TO SEE YOUR DOCTOR
Asthma or possibly heart failure may be the cause of your symptoms.

● If you smoke, give up immediately.

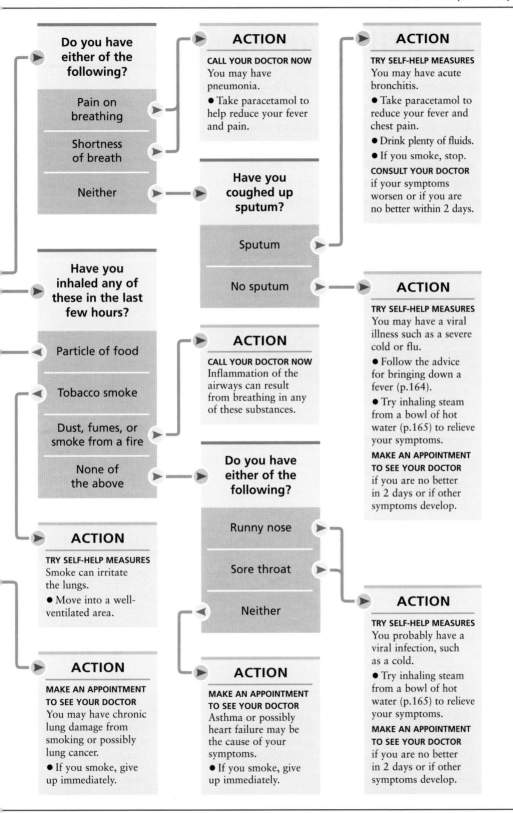

Coughing (children)

◄ **For adults and children over 12, see p.106**
Coughing is a normal reaction to irritation in the throat or lungs. Most coughs are due to minor infections of the nose and/or throat, but a sudden onset of coughing may be caused by choking. Coughing is unusual in babies under 6 months old and may indicate a serious lung infection.

Danger signs
Call an ambulance if your child is coughing and has any of the following symptoms:
- Blue-tinged lips or tongue.
- Abnormal drowsiness.
- Inability to talk or produce sounds.
- Inability to drink.

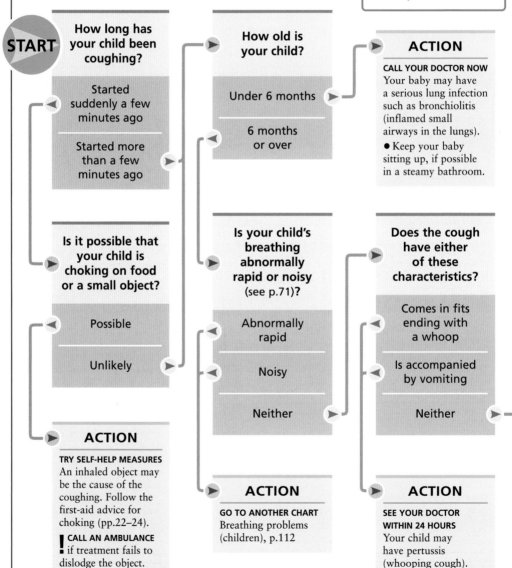

START

How long has your child been coughing?

Started suddenly a few minutes ago

Started more than a few minutes ago

How old is your child?

Under 6 months

6 months or over

ACTION

CALL YOUR DOCTOR NOW
Your baby may have a serious lung infection such as bronchiolitis (inflamed small airways in the lungs).
● Keep your baby sitting up, if possible in a steamy bathroom.

Is it possible that your child is choking on food or a small object?

Possible

Unlikely

Is your child's breathing abnormally rapid or noisy (see p.71)?

Abnormally rapid

Noisy

Neither

Does the cough have either of these characteristics?

Comes in fits ending with a whoop

Is accompanied by vomiting

Neither

ACTION

TRY SELF-HELP MEASURES
An inhaled object may be the cause of the coughing. Follow the first-aid advice for choking (pp.22–24).

❚ **CALL AN AMBULANCE** if treatment fails to dislodge the object.

ACTION

GO TO ANOTHER CHART
Breathing problems (children), p.112

ACTION

SEE YOUR DOCTOR WITHIN 24 HOURS
Your child may have pertussis (whooping cough).

Does your child have a runny nose?

Most of the time or very often ▶

Has developed a runny nose within the past few days ▶

No runny nose ◀

When does the coughing occur?

Mainly at night ◀

After exercise ◀

When out in the cold ◀

None of the above ▶

Are there smokers in the home or might your child have been smoking?

Smokers in the home ▶

Child might smoke ▶

Neither ◀

Does your child have a fever – a temperature of 38°C (100°F) or above?

Fever ▶

No fever ▶

ACTION

MAKE AN APPOINTMENT TO SEE YOUR DOCTOR
Your child may have an allergy or possibly enlarged adenoids.

ACTION

TRY SELF-HELP MEASURES
Your child probably has a viral illness, such as a cold or flu.
● Follow the advice for bringing down a fever (p.164).
●Try inhaling steam from a bowl of hot water (p.165) or sitting in a steamy bathroom.
CONSULT YOUR DOCTOR if symptoms worsen, if your child is no better in 2 days, or if other symptoms develop.

ACTION

TRY SELF-HELP MEASURES
Your child probably has a cold.
●Try inhaling steam from a bowl of hot water (p.165) or sitting in a steamy bathroom.
CONSULT YOUR DOCTOR if symptoms worsen, if your child is no better in 2 days, or if other symptoms develop.

ACTION

TRY SELF-HELP MEASURES
Your child's cough may be a response to being in a smoky atmosphere or to his or her own smoking.
● Make sure that no one smokes in the house and avoid taking your child into a smoky atmosphere.
● If you suspect that your child may be smoking, encourage him or her to stop.

ACTION

SEE YOUR DOCTOR WITHIN 24 HOURS
Your child's symptoms may be due to asthma.
● Discourage your child from activities that provoke coughing.
● Avoid unnecessary exposure to dust, pollen, or animal fur.

ACTION

SEE YOUR DOCTOR WITHIN 24 HOURS
if you cannot identify a possible cause for your child's cough from this chart.

Shortness of breath (adults)

For children under 12, see p.112 ▶

Feeling short of breath is to be expected after strenuous exercise. Breathing should return to normal after resting. If you are short of breath at rest or after normal activities, such as getting dressed, you should consult your doctor because your symptom may be due to a serious heart or lung disorder.

❗ Danger signs

Call an ambulance if either you or someone you are with has one or both of the following symptoms:
● Sudden and severe shortness of breath.
● Blue-tinged lips.
While waiting for medical help, loosen any restricting clothing and help the person to sit upright.

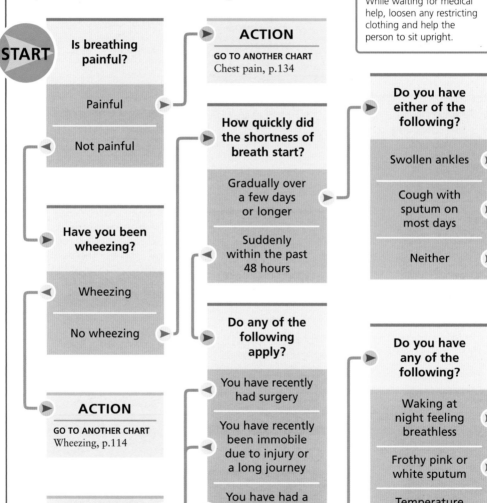

START

Is breathing painful?

Painful ▶

Not painful

Have you been wheezing?

Wheezing

No wheezing ▶

ACTION
GO TO ANOTHER CHART
Wheezing, p.114

ACTION ◀
❗ CALL AN AMBULANCE
You may have a pulmonary embolism (blood clot in the lung).

ACTION
GO TO ANOTHER CHART
Chest pain, p.134

How quickly did the shortness of breath start?

Gradually over a few days or longer

Suddenly within the past 48 hours ◀

Do any of the following apply?

You have recently had surgery

You have recently been immobile due to injury or a long journey

You have had a baby within the past 2 weeks

None of the above ▶

Do you have either of the following?

Swollen ankles ▶

Cough with sputum on most days ▶

Neither ▶

Do you have any of the following?

Waking at night feeling breathless ▶

Frothy pink or white sputum ▶

Temperature of 38°C (100°F) or above ▶

None of the above ▶

ACTION

SEE YOUR DOCTOR WITHIN 24 HOURS
You may have chronic heart failure, in which fluid accumulates in the lungs and tissues.
● If you smoke, stop.
● Avoid strenuous exercise and stressful situations.

ACTION

MAKE AN APPOINTMENT TO SEE YOUR DOCTOR
You may have lung disease caused by inhaling damaging dusts or gases.

ACTION

MAKE AN APPOINTMENT TO SEE YOUR DOCTOR
You may have inflammation of the lungs due to an allergy.

Do you have, or have you ever had, regular exposure to or contact with the following?

Dust or fumes ▷

Grain crops, caged birds, or animals ▷

Neither ▷

ACTION

MAKE AN APPOINTMENT TO SEE YOUR DOCTOR
You may have chronic lung damage from smoking.
● If you smoke, stop.
● Avoid exposure to smoke, pollution, dust, dampness, and cold.
● Take gentle exercise.

ACTION

SEE YOUR DOCTOR WITHIN 24 HOURS
You may be anaemic, but a blood test will be needed to confirm the diagnosis.
● Get plenty of rest.

Did the shortness of breath start straight after a stressful event?

Yes ◁

No ▷

Do you have any of the following?

Faintness or fainting ▷

Paler skin than normal ▷

Undue tiredness ▷

None of the above ◁

ACTION

CALL YOUR DOCTOR NOW
You may have fluid on the lungs (pulmonary oedema) caused by acute heart failure.

ACTION

CALL YOUR DOCTOR NOW
You may have a lung infection, such as pneumonia, especially if you also have a cough.
● Take paracetamol to reduce fever.

ACTION

CALL YOUR DOCTOR NOW
You may have had a panic attack, but this needs to be confirmed by a doctor.
● If you have had such attacks before, rebreathing into a bag may relieve symptoms (p.168).

ACTION

SEE YOUR DOCTOR WITHIN 24 HOURS
if you cannot identify a possible cause for your shortness of breath from this chart.

Breathing problems (children)

◀ **For adults and children over 12, see p.110**
Noisy or rapid breathing and shortness of breath indicate breathing problems. Such problems may not be obvious in children because they may simply avoid exertion. A child with severe difficulty breathing needs urgent hospital treatment. Breathing problems that occur suddenly also need immediate attention.

Danger signs
Call an ambulance if your child's breathing rate is excessively rapid (see advice on checking your child's breathing rate, p.71) and if breathing problems are accompanied by any of the following symptoms:
● Blue-tinged lips or tongue.
● Abnormal drowsiness.
● Inability to swallow, talk, or produce sounds.

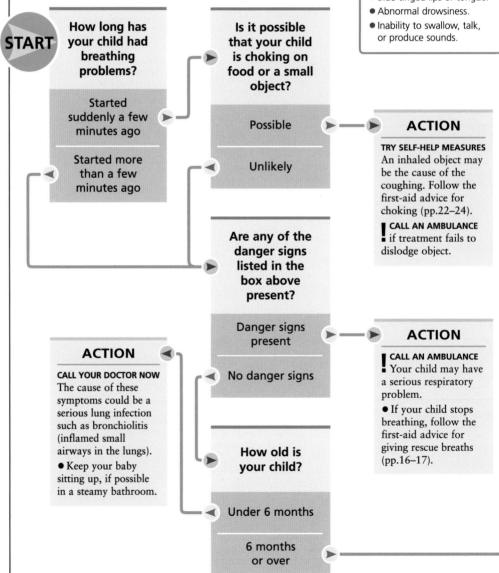

START

How long has your child had breathing problems?

Started suddenly a few minutes ago

Started more than a few minutes ago

Is it possible that your child is choking on food or a small object?

Possible

Unlikely

ACTION

TRY SELF-HELP MEASURES An inhaled object may be the cause of the coughing. Follow the first-aid advice for choking (pp.22–24).

! **CALL AN AMBULANCE** if treatment fails to dislodge object.

Are any of the danger signs listed in the box above present?

Danger signs present

No danger signs

ACTION

! **CALL AN AMBULANCE** Your child may have a serious respiratory problem.
● If your child stops breathing, follow the first-aid advice for giving rescue breaths (pp.16–17).

ACTION

CALL YOUR DOCTOR NOW The cause of these symptoms could be a serious lung infection such as bronchiolitis (inflamed small airways in the lungs).
● Keep your baby sitting up, if possible in a steamy bathroom.

How old is your child?

Under 6 months

6 months or over

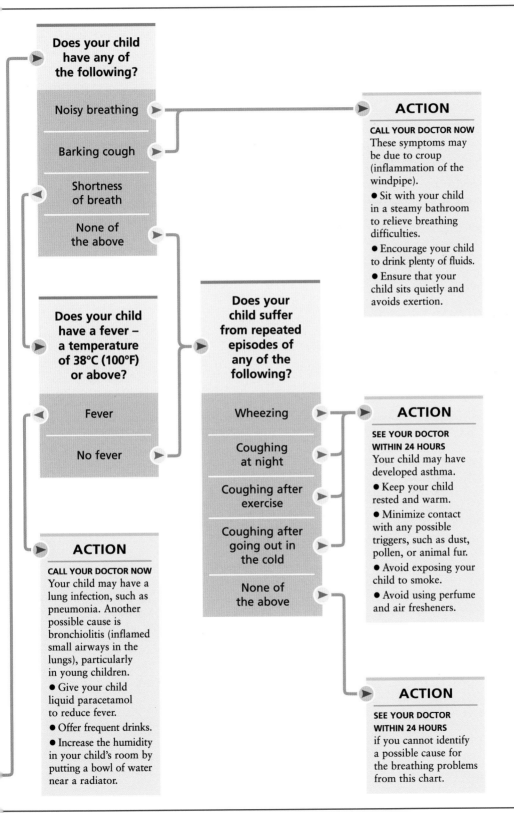

Does your child have any of the following?

Noisy breathing

Barking cough

Shortness of breath

None of the above

Does your child have a fever – a temperature of 38°C (100°F) or above?

Fever

No fever

Does your child suffer from repeated episodes of any of the following?

Wheezing

Coughing at night

Coughing after exercise

Coughing after going out in the cold

None of the above

ACTION

CALL YOUR DOCTOR NOW
These symptoms may be due to croup (inflammation of the windpipe).
● Sit with your child in a steamy bathroom to relieve breathing difficulties.
● Encourage your child to drink plenty of fluids.
● Ensure that your child sits quietly and avoids exertion.

ACTION

SEE YOUR DOCTOR WITHIN 24 HOURS
Your child may have developed asthma.
● Keep your child rested and warm.
● Minimize contact with any possible triggers, such as dust, pollen, or animal fur.
● Avoid exposing your child to smoke.
● Avoid using perfume and air fresheners.

ACTION

CALL YOUR DOCTOR NOW
Your child may have a lung infection, such as pneumonia. Another possible cause is bronchiolitis (inflamed small airways in the lungs), particularly in young children.
● Give your child liquid paracetamol to reduce fever.
● Offer frequent drinks.
● Increase the humidity in your child's room by putting a bowl of water near a radiator.

ACTION

SEE YOUR DOCTOR WITHIN 24 HOURS
if you cannot identify a possible cause for the breathing problems from this chart.

Wheezing

◄ For children under 12, see p.112

A whistling or rasping sound on exhaling occurs when the air passages become narrowed. The most common causes are inflammation due to infection, asthma, or inhaled dust. In rare cases, a narrowing of the airways may be due to a tumour. If you have persistent wheezing, you should see your doctor.

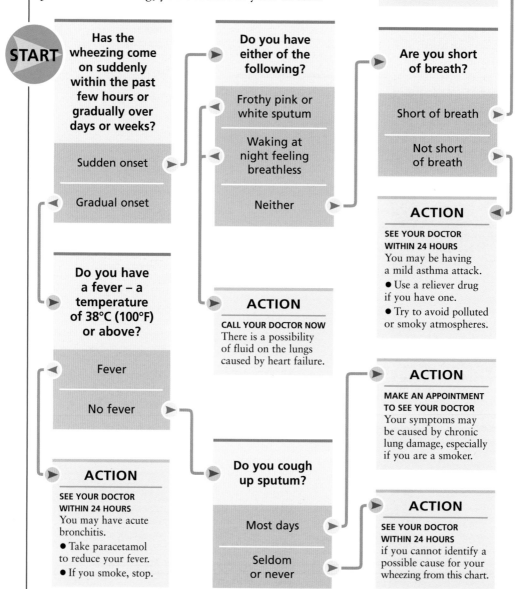

ACTION ◄

CALL YOUR DOCTOR NOW
You could be having an asthma attack.
• If you have a reliever inhaler, use it now.
• Stay calm and sit in a comfortable position.

START Has the wheezing come on suddenly within the past few hours or gradually over days or weeks?

Sudden onset ►

Gradual onset ◄

Do you have either of the following?

Frothy pink or white sputum ◄

Waking at night feeling breathless ◄

Neither ►

Are you short of breath?

Short of breath ►

Not short of breath ►

ACTION ◄

SEE YOUR DOCTOR WITHIN 24 HOURS
You may be having a mild asthma attack.
• Use a reliever drug if you have one.
• Try to avoid polluted or smoky atmospheres.

Do you have a fever – a temperature of 38°C (100°F) or above?

Fever ◄

No fever ►

ACTION ►

CALL YOUR DOCTOR NOW
There is a possibility of fluid on the lungs caused by heart failure.

ACTION ►

MAKE AN APPOINTMENT TO SEE YOUR DOCTOR
Your symptoms may be caused by chronic lung damage, especially if you are a smoker.

ACTION ►

SEE YOUR DOCTOR WITHIN 24 HOURS
You may have acute bronchitis.
• Take paracetamol to reduce your fever.
• If you smoke, stop.

Do you cough up sputum?

Most days ►

Seldom or never ►

ACTION ►

SEE YOUR DOCTOR WITHIN 24 HOURS
if you cannot identify a possible cause for your wheezing from this chart.

Difficulty swallowing

Any difficulty swallowing is usually the result of a sore throat due to infection. Self-treatment should ease the soreness and allow normal swallowing. However, persistent difficulty with swallowing may be due to a disorder of the stomach or oesophagus, the tube connecting the throat to the stomach, and should be investigated by your doctor.

START

Is your throat sore?

- Sore
- Not sore

Is it possible that you have swallowed something sharp, such as a fish bone?

- Possible
- Unlikely

ACTION

GO TO ANOTHER CHART
Sore throat, p.103

ACTION

CALL YOUR DOCTOR NOW
Something may have either scratched your throat or become lodged in it.

Which of the following applies?

- Food seems to stick high up in the chest
- You have a feeling of something being stuck in the throat
- Neither

ACTION

MAKE AN APPOINTMENT TO SEE YOUR DOCTOR
Anxiety disorders may be a cause of this type of difficulty with swallowing.

ACTION

MAKE AN APPOINTMENT TO SEE YOUR DOCTOR
if you cannot identify a possible cause for your difficulty swallowing from this chart.

Do you get a burning pain in the centre of the chest in either of these situations?

- When you bend forwards
- When you lie down
- Neither

ACTION

MAKE AN APPOINTMENT TO SEE YOUR DOCTOR
You probably have an inflamed oesophagus due to acid reflux.

Does either of the following apply?

- The swallowing difficulty is getting worse
- You have lost weight
- Neither

ACTION

SEE YOUR DOCTOR WITHIN 24 HOURS
You may have a narrowed oesophagus caused by acid reflux, but cancer of the oesophagus is possible.

Vomiting (adults)

For children under 12, see p.118 ►
Irritation or inflammation of the digestive tract is
the most common cause of vomiting. It may also
be triggered by conditions affecting the brain or
by an inner-ear disorder, or it can be a side effect
of medication. If you often suffer from episodes of
vomiting, you should consult your doctor.

Danger signs
Call an ambulance if your
vomit contains blood, which
may appear in any of the
following forms:
- Bright red streaks.
- Black material that
  resembles coffee grounds.
- Blood clots.

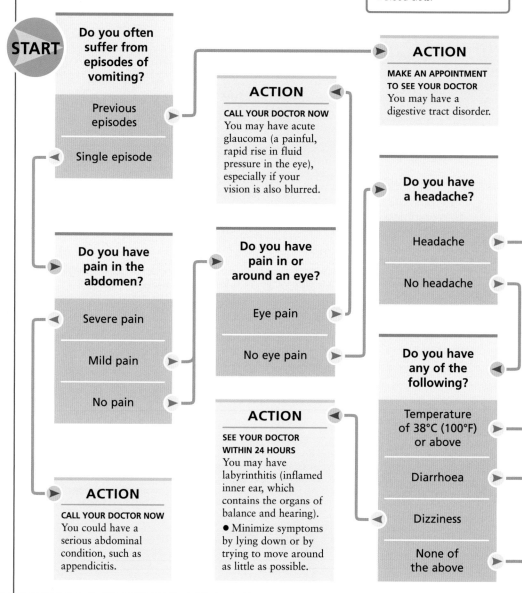

START

Do you often suffer from episodes of vomiting?

- Previous episodes
- Single episode

Do you have pain in the abdomen?

- Severe pain
- Mild pain
- No pain

ACTION

CALL YOUR DOCTOR NOW
You could have a
serious abdominal
condition, such as
appendicitis.

Do you have pain in or around an eye?

- Eye pain
- No eye pain

ACTION

CALL YOUR DOCTOR NOW
You may have acute
glaucoma (a painful,
rapid rise in fluid
pressure in the eye),
especially if your
vision is also blurred.

ACTION

**SEE YOUR DOCTOR
WITHIN 24 HOURS**
You may have
labyrinthitis (inflamed
inner ear, which
contains the organs of
balance and hearing).
- Minimize symptoms
by lying down or by
trying to move around
as little as possible.

ACTION

**MAKE AN APPOINTMENT
TO SEE YOUR DOCTOR**
You may have a
digestive tract disorder.

Do you have a headache?

- Headache
- No headache

Do you have any of the following?

- Temperature of 38°C (100°F) or above
- Diarrhoea
- Dizziness
- None of the above

ⓘ Vomiting and medications

If you are taking any oral medication, including oral contraceptives, an episode of vomiting may reduce the effectiveness of the drug because your body cannot absorb the active ingredients. If you use oral contraceptives, you will need to use an additional form of contraception such as condoms for some time after the vomiting has stopped. Follow the instructions provided with the oral contraceptives or consult your doctor if you are not sure what to do. You should also see your doctor if you are taking any other prescribed medicine and have been vomiting.

Have you eaten or drunk any of the following?

An unusually large or rich meal

A large amount of alcohol

Food that may have been contaminated

None of the above

ACTION

TRY SELF-HELP MEASURES
You probably have gastritis (inflammation of the stomach lining).

● Take over-the-counter antacids to neutralize the acid in the stomach.
● Eat small meals at regular intervals.
● Stop drinking alcohol until you are better.
● If you smoke, stop.

CONSULT YOUR DOCTOR
if you are no better in 2 days or if other symptoms develop.

ACTION

GO TO ANOTHER CHART
Headache, p.84

ACTION

TRY SELF-HELP MEASURES
You may have food poisoning.

● Follow the advice for preventing dehydration (p.165).

CONSULT YOUR DOCTOR
if you are no better in 2 days or if other symptoms develop.

Are you taking any medication?

Medication

No medication

ACTION

TRY SELF-HELP MEASURES
You may have a case of gastroenteritis.

● Follow the advice for preventing dehydration (p.165).

CONSULT YOUR DOCTOR
if you are no better in 2 days or if other symptoms develop.

ACTION

SEE YOUR DOCTOR WITHIN 24 HOURS
Your symptoms may be a side effect of the medication.

● Stop taking any over-the-counter medicines but continue to take prescribed medication unless advised to stop by your doctor.

ACTION

SEE YOUR DOCTOR WITHIN 24 HOURS
if you cannot identify a possible cause for your vomiting from this chart.

Vomiting (children)

◀ **For adults and children over 12, see p.116**

Children vomit as a result of many illnesses, including ear infections and urinary and digestive tract disorders. Anxiety or excitement may also cause vomiting. Rarely, vomiting may be due to an infection or injury to the brain. If vomiting is persistent, you should consult your doctor urgently.

Danger signs

Call an ambulance if your child's vomiting is accompanied by any of the following symptoms:

- Greenish-yellow vomit.
- Abdominal pain for 4 hours.
- Flat, dark-red or purple spots that do not fade when pressed.
- Refusal to drink or feed (in babies) for over 6 hours.
- Abnormal drowsiness.
- Sunken eyes.
- Dry tongue.
- Passing no urine during the day for 3 hours (if child is under 1 year old) or 6 hours (in an older child).
- Black or bloodstained faeces.

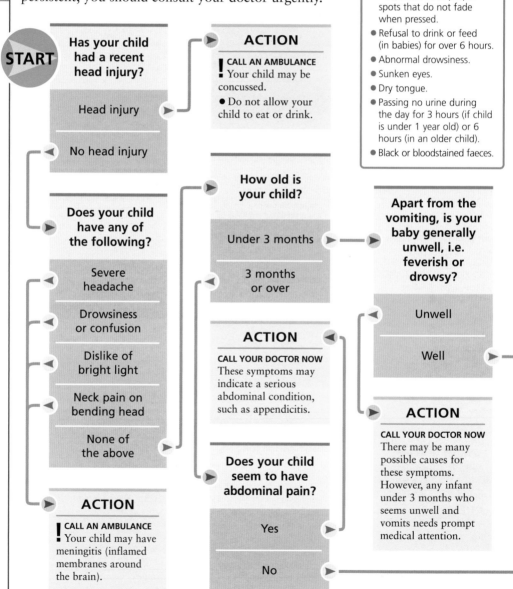

START

Has your child had a recent head injury?

Head injury ▶

ACTION
! **CALL AN AMBULANCE**
Your child may be concussed.
- Do not allow your child to eat or drink.

No head injury

Does your child have any of the following?

- Severe headache
- Drowsiness or confusion
- Dislike of bright light
- Neck pain on bending head
- None of the above ▶

ACTION
! **CALL AN AMBULANCE**
Your child may have meningitis (inflamed membranes around the brain).

How old is your child?

Under 3 months ▶

3 months or over

ACTION
CALL YOUR DOCTOR NOW
These symptoms may indicate a serious abdominal condition, such as appendicitis.

Does your child seem to have abdominal pain?

Yes ▶

No ▶

Apart from the vomiting, is your baby generally unwell, i.e. feverish or drowsy?

Unwell

Well ▶

ACTION
CALL YOUR DOCTOR NOW
There may be many possible causes for these symptoms. However, any infant under 3 months who seems unwell and vomits needs prompt medical attention.

What are the characteristics of the vomiting?

Frequent and effortless after feeds

Forceful after several feeds

Occasional, not associated with feeding

ACTION

TRY SELF-HELP MEASURES
Babies often vomit for no particular reason, and this is no cause for concern if your baby seems generally well and is gaining weight.
● Be sure to wind your baby after each feed.
CONSULT YOUR DOCTOR
if your baby seems unwell or vomits often.

ACTION

CALL YOUR DOCTOR NOW
Your child may have a lung infection such as pertussis (whooping cough), bronchiolitis, or pneumonia.

Did vomiting follow violent coughing?

Followed coughing

No coughing

ACTION

SEE YOUR DOCTOR WITHIN 24 HOURS
This type of vomiting in an infant may be the result of a digestive tract problem, such as pyloric stenosis, in which the stomach outlet becomes abnormally narrowed.

Does your child have diarrhoea?

Diarrhoea

No diarrhoea

Does your child have any of the following?

Pain on passing urine

Renewed bedwetting or daytime "accidents"

Temperature of 38°C (100°F) or above

None of the above

ACTION

SEE YOUR DOCTOR WITHIN 24 HOURS
if you cannot identify a possible cause for your child's vomiting from this chart.

ACTION

TRY SELF-HELP MEASURES
This type of vomiting is rarely serious and has several possible causes.
● Always wind your baby after feeding.
CONSULT YOUR DOCTOR
if your infant seems unwell or is failing to gain weight.

ACTION

CALL YOUR DOCTOR NOW
if your child is under 6 months old. He or she may have a case of gastroenteritis.
● Make sure older children drink plenty of clear fluids.
CONSULT YOUR DOCTOR
if your child is no better within 24 hours or if any other symptoms develop.

ACTION

SEE YOUR DOCTOR WITHIN 24 HOURS
Your child may have a urinary tract infection.
● Give plenty of fluids to drink.

ACTION

SEE YOUR DOCTOR WITHIN 24 HOURS
Your child may have an infection such as acute otitis media (an infection of the middle ear) or a urinary tract infection.
● Give your child liquid paracetamol to relieve pain and fever.

Abdominal pain (adults)

For children under 12, see p.124 ▶
Mild abdominal pain is often due to a stomach or
bowel upset that will clear up without treatment.
However, severe or persistent abdominal pain,
especially if it is accompanied by other symptoms,
may indicate a more serious problem that should
be investigated by your doctor.

Danger signs
Call an ambulance if you
have severe abdominal pain
that lasts for longer than
4 hours and is associated
with any of the following
additional symptoms:
- Vomiting.
- Fever.
- Swollen or tender abdomen.
- Feeling faint, drowsy, or
confused.
- Blood in the urine or faeces.

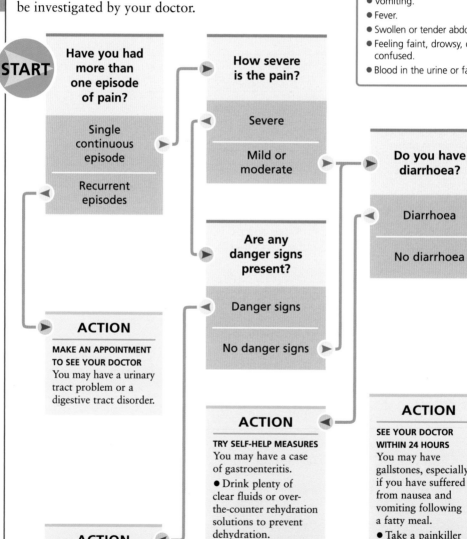

START

Have you had more than one episode of pain?

Single continuous episode

Recurrent episodes

How severe is the pain?

Severe

Mild or moderate

Are any danger signs present?

Danger signs

No danger signs

Do you have diarrhoea?

Diarrhoea

No diarrhoea

ACTION

MAKE AN APPOINTMENT TO SEE YOUR DOCTOR
You may have a urinary
tract problem or a
digestive tract disorder.

ACTION

TRY SELF-HELP MEASURES
You may have a case
of gastroenteritis.
- Drink plenty of
clear fluids or over-
the-counter rehydration
solutions to prevent
dehydration.

CONSULT YOUR DOCTOR
if you are no better
in 2 days or if other
symptoms develop.

ACTION

**SEE YOUR DOCTOR
WITHIN 24 HOURS**
You may have
gallstones, especially
if you have suffered
from nausea and
vomiting following
a fatty meal.
- Take a painkiller
such as paracetamol
to relieve symptoms.
- Avoid eating foods
that are high in fat.

ACTION

! CALL AN AMBULANCE
You may have
appendicitis.

ACTION

CALL YOUR DOCTOR NOW
You may have kidney
stones, especially if you
have been vomiting.
● Drink plenty of
fluids to flush the
stones into the urine.
● Save any urine you
pass, particularly if
you pass a stone.
● Take paracetamol to
relieve the discomfort.

What kind of pain have you been experiencing?

Pain that starts in the back and may move to the groin

Pain in the centre of the upper abdomen

Pain in the upper right abdomen that may spread to the back

Pain mainly below the waist

None of the above

ACTION

**SEE YOUR DOCTOR
WITHIN 24 HOURS**
if you cannot identify
a possible cause for
your abdominal pain
from this chart.

Do any of the following apply?

Pain is related to eating

Pain is relieved by antacids

Pain comes on when lying or bending over

None of the above

Do you have either of the following?

Pain on passing urine

Passing urine more often than usual

Neither

Are you female or male?

Female

Male

ACTION

**MAKE AN APPOINTMENT
TO SEE YOUR DOCTOR**
You may have
nonulcer dyspepsia (a
recurrent and persistent
form of indigestion) or
gastro-oesophageal
reflux, in which acid
from the stomach is
regurgitated into the
oesophagus.
● Eat small meals at
regular intervals.
● Avoid eating shortly
before going to bed.
● Reduce your intake of
alcohol, coffee, and tea.
● If you smoke, stop.

ACTION

GO TO ANOTHER CHART
Chest pain, p.134

ACTION

**SEE YOUR DOCTOR
WITHIN 24 HOURS**
You may have cystitis
or a urine infection
that has spread to one
or both kidneys.
● For both conditions,
take a painkiller such
as paracetamol.
● Drink 500 ml (1 pt)
of fluid every hour for
4 hours.
● Drinking cranberry
juice may relieve the
burning sensation.

ACTION

GO TO ANOTHER CHART
Abdominal pain
(women), p.122

Abdominal pain (women)

◀ First refer to abdominal pain, p.120

Several disorders specific to women can cause discomfort or pain in the lower abdomen. Many of these conditions are related to the reproductive tract (ovaries, uterus, or fallopian tubes) or to pregnancy. Abdominal pain that occurs during pregnancy should always be taken seriously.

❗ Abdominal pain in pregnancy

Intermittent, mild abdominal pains are common throughout pregnancy due to stretching of the muscles and ligaments of the abdomen. Abdominal pain that occurs in early pregnancy can be due to complications, such as miscarriage or an ectopic pregnancy. In later pregnancy, pain is most commonly caused by the onset of labour. Rarely, partial separation of the placenta from the wall of the uterus may occur.

● If you develop severe pain, call your doctor at once.

START

Do you have pain when you pass urine?

Yes ▶

No ▶

ACTION

SEE YOUR DOCTOR WITHIN 24 HOURS
You may have cystitis.

● Take a painkiller such as paracetamol.

● Drink 500 ml (1 pt) of fluid every hour for 4 hours.

● Drinking cranberry juice may help relieve the burning sensation.

Are you pregnant?

More than 14 weeks pregnant

Less than 14 weeks pregnant

Do not think so ▶

ACTION

CALL YOUR DOCTOR NOW
You could be having a late miscarriage or placental abruption (separation of the placenta from the wall of the uterus).

● Rest in bed until you receive medical advice.

ACTION

CALL YOUR DOCTOR NOW
Pain at this stage may indicate a threatened miscarriage or an ectopic pregnancy.

● Rest in bed until you receive medical advice.

Have you had sexual intercourse in the past 3 months?

Yes

No ▶

Did your last period occur at the time you expected?

On time ▶

Missed or late ▶

Do you have any of the following?

Abnormal vaginal discharge

Fever

None of the above

ACTION

SEE YOUR DOCTOR WITHIN 24 HOURS
You may have pelvic inflammatory disease, in which there is an infection in the reproductive organs.
• Your partner may also need to have tests for infection.

Do you have an intrauterine contraceptive device (IUD)?

IUD

No IUD

Is the pain related to your menstrual cycle?

Occurs just before and/or during a period

Occurs briefly in midcycle

Unrelated

Have you been through the menopause?

Premenopausal

Postmenopausal

ACTION

MAKE AN APPOINTMENT TO SEE YOUR DOCTOR
This particular form of contraception often causes increased period pain, particularly for the first few cycles after it has been inserted.

ACTION

MAKE AN APPOINTMENT TO SEE YOUR DOCTOR
Some women regularly have pain associated with their ovulation. However, other possible causes do need to be ruled out.

ACTION

CALL YOUR DOCTOR NOW
There is a possibility of an ectopic pregnancy.
• Rest in bed until you receive medical advice.

ACTION

MAKE AN APPOINTMENT TO SEE YOUR DOCTOR
if you cannot identify a possible cause for your lower abdominal pain from this chart.

ACTION

GO TO ANOTHER CHART
Painful periods, p.156

Abdominal pain (children)

◀ For adults and children over 12, see p.120

Many children suffer from abdominal pain at some time, and some children have recurrent episodes. Usually, the cause is not serious, and the pain subsides in a few hours without treatment. In rare cases, abdominal pain is a symptom of a serious disorder that requires prompt medical attention.

Danger signs

Call an ambulance if your child's abdominal pain is accompanied by any of the following symptoms:
- Greenish-yellow vomit.
- Pain in the groin or scrotum.
- Blood in the faeces.
- Pain has been continuous for more than 4 hours.

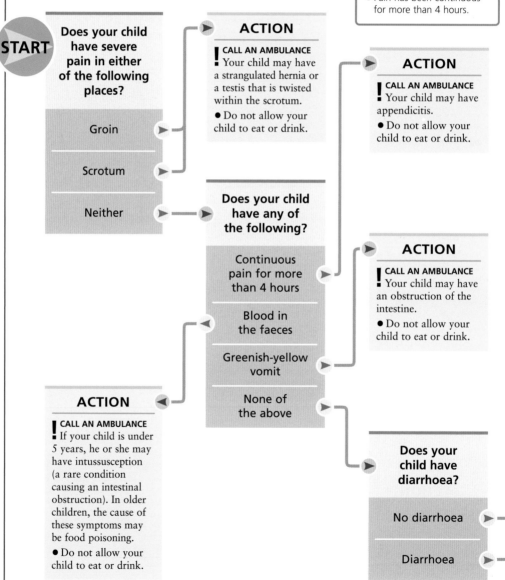

START

Does your child have severe pain in either of the following places?

Groin

Scrotum

Neither

ACTION

! CALL AN AMBULANCE
■ Your child may have a strangulated hernia or a testis that is twisted within the scrotum.
● Do not allow your child to eat or drink.

ACTION

! CALL AN AMBULANCE
■ Your child may have appendicitis.
● Do not allow your child to eat or drink.

Does your child have any of the following?

Continuous pain for more than 4 hours

Blood in the faeces

Greenish-yellow vomit

None of the above

ACTION

! CALL AN AMBULANCE
■ Your child may have an obstruction of the intestine.
● Do not allow your child to eat or drink.

ACTION

! CALL AN AMBULANCE
■ If your child is under 5 years, he or she may have intussusception (a rare condition causing an intestinal obstruction). In older children, the cause of these symptoms may be food poisoning.
● Do not allow your child to eat or drink.

Does your child have diarrhoea?

No diarrhoea

Diarrhoea

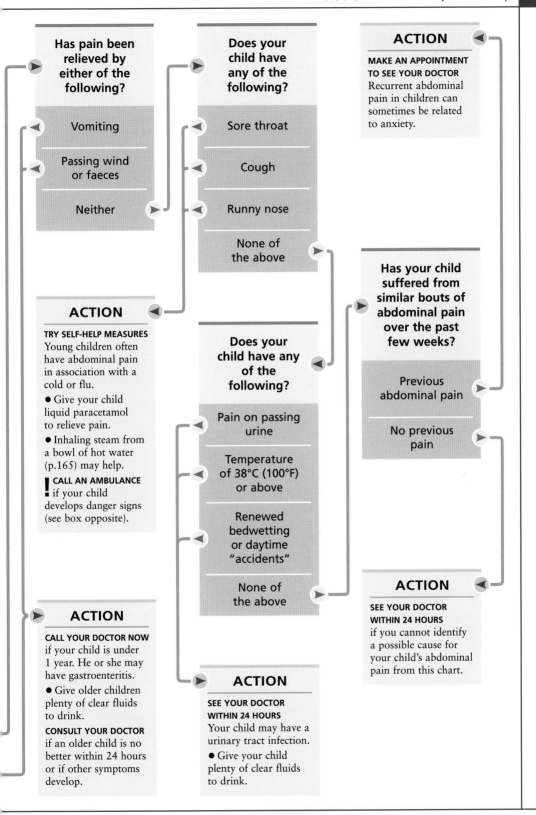

Has pain been relieved by either of the following?

- Vomiting
- Passing wind or faeces
- Neither

Does your child have any of the following?

- Sore throat
- Cough
- Runny nose
- None of the above

ACTION

MAKE AN APPOINTMENT TO SEE YOUR DOCTOR Recurrent abdominal pain in children can sometimes be related to anxiety.

ACTION

TRY SELF-HELP MEASURES Young children often have abdominal pain in association with a cold or flu.

- Give your child liquid paracetamol to relieve pain.
- Inhaling steam from a bowl of hot water (p.165) may help.

! CALL AN AMBULANCE if your child develops danger signs (see box opposite).

Does your child have any of the following?

- Pain on passing urine
- Temperature of 38°C (100°F) or above
- Renewed bedwetting or daytime "accidents"
- None of the above

Has your child suffered from similar bouts of abdominal pain over the past few weeks?

- Previous abdominal pain
- No previous pain

ACTION

CALL YOUR DOCTOR NOW if your child is under 1 year. He or she may have gastroenteritis.

- Give older children plenty of clear fluids to drink.

CONSULT YOUR DOCTOR if an older child is no better within 24 hours or if other symptoms develop.

ACTION

SEE YOUR DOCTOR WITHIN 24 HOURS if you cannot identify a possible cause for your child's abdominal pain from this chart.

ACTION

SEE YOUR DOCTOR WITHIN 24 HOURS Your child may have a urinary tract infection.

- Give your child plenty of clear fluids to drink.

Swollen abdomen

Enlargement of the abdomen is usually due to weight gain or poor muscle tone from lack of exercise. A swollen abdomen may also result from a disorder of either the digestive system or the urinary system. If you have abdominal swelling that has come on rapidly, you should consult your doctor irrespective of any other symptoms you may have.

ACTION

GO TO ANOTHER CHART
Abdominal pain
(adults), p.120, or
Abdominal pain
(children), p.124

START

How long has your abdomen been swollen?

Less than 24 hours

Longer than 24 hours

Do you have abdominal pain?

Severe pain

Mild pain

No pain

ACTION

MAKE AN APPOINTMENT
TO SEE YOUR DOCTOR
You may be suffering
from excessive wind or
constipation, possibly
due to irritable bowel
syndrome.

Is the pain relieved by passing wind or having a bowel movement?

Relieved

Unrelieved

ACTION

TRY SELF-HELP MEASURES
A swollen abdomen
may be the the first
sign of an unsuspected
pregnancy, especially
if you have been using
contraception or if
your periods tend to
be irregular.
● If you think that
you might be pregnant,
carry out a home
pregnancy test.

Do any of the following apply?

Your ankles are swollen

You could be pregnant

You have difficulty passing urine

You pass only small volumes of urine

None of the above

ACTION

GO TO ANOTHER CHART
Swollen ankles, p.148

ACTION

MAKE AN APPOINTMENT
TO SEE YOUR DOCTOR
if you cannot identify
a possible cause for
your swollen abdomen
from this chart.

ACTION

SEE YOUR DOCTOR
WITHIN 24 HOURS
The swelling could be
due to an abnormally
full bladder caused
by a blockage at the
bladder outlet.

Anal and rectal problems

The anus is the opening of the lower large intestine (rectum) to the outside. Discomfort during bowel movements may be due to a disorder of the rectum, the anus, or the skin around the anus. Rectal or anal bleeding is often due to haemorrhoids but can also be an early symptom of cancer. Consult your doctor if you have any bleeding or persistent discomfort.

START

Have you noticed bleeding from the anus?

Bleeding

No bleeding

Do you have either of the following?

Pain in or around the anus or rectum

Sore area in the crease above the anus

Neither

ACTION

SEE YOUR DOCTOR WITHIN 24 HOURS
You may have a pilonidal sinus (small pit at the top of this crease, which can result in an abscess).
● Soak the affected area in warm water.

ACTION

SEE YOUR DOCTOR WITHIN 24 HOURS
Although haemorrhoids (piles) are a likely cause, there is a slight possibility of cancer of the colon, rectum, or anus that needs to be excluded.

Do you have itching around the anus?

Itching

No itching

Do you have small, irregular, fleshy lumps around the anus?

Yes

No

ACTION

MAKE AN APPOINTMENT TO SEE YOUR DOCTOR
You may have a threadworm infestation.

Do you have either of the following?

White "threads" in your faeces

Itching is worse in bed at night

Neither

ACTION

TRY SELF-HELP MEASURES
You may have haemorrhoids (piles), but itching can occur for no obvious reason.
● Try using an over-the-counter haemorrhoid preparation to relieve the itching.
CONSULT YOUR DOCTOR if the itching continues for more than 3 days.

ACTION

MAKE AN APPOINTMENT TO SEE YOUR DOCTOR
It is possible that you have genital warts.

ACTION

MAKE AN APPOINTMENT TO SEE YOUR DOCTOR
if you cannot identify a possible cause for your anal or rectal problem from this chart.

Diarrhoea (adults)

For children under 12 years, see p.130 ▶
Diarrhoea is the frequent passing of abnormally loose or watery faeces, and is usually a result of infection. However, persistent diarrhoea may be caused by a serious gastrointestinal disorder. You should consult your doctor if diarrhoea continues for more than 2 days or if it recurs.

! Dehydration

A person with bad diarrhoea can become dehydrated if fluids are not replaced quickly enough. The symptoms of dehydration include confusion or drowsiness, a dry mouth, loss of elasticity in the skin, and failure to pass urine for several hours. Elderly people are particularly at risk. Follow the advice for preventing dehydration on p.165, but seek urgent medical help if a person has severe symptoms.

START

Have you noticed blood in your faeces?

- Blood
- No blood ▶

Have you had several bouts of diarrhoea over the past few weeks?

- Yes ▶
- No ◀

Has the diarrhoea been alternating with bouts of constipation?

- Constipation and diarrhoea ◀
- Diarrhoea alone ▶

ACTION

SEE YOUR DOCTOR WITHIN 24 HOURS
You may have an intestinal infection, such as amoebiasis, or ulcerative colitis (ulceration of the rectum and colon). However, the slight possibility of cancer of the colon or rectum needs to be excluded.

ACTION

MAKE AN APPOINTMENT TO SEE YOUR DOCTOR
You probably have irritable bowel syndrome, especially if you have suffered abdominal pain and excessive wind. However, the slight possibility of cancer of the colon or rectum needs to be excluded.
- Avoid large meals, spicy, fried, and fatty foods, and milk products.
- Cut down on coffee, tea, cola, and beer.

ACTION

TRY SELF-HELP MEASURES
You may have food poisoning.
- Follow the advice for preventing dehydration (p.165).

CONSULT YOUR DOCTOR if you are no better in 2 days or if any other symptoms develop.

Have you recently consumed food or water that may have been contaminated?

- Possible ▶
- Unlikely ▶

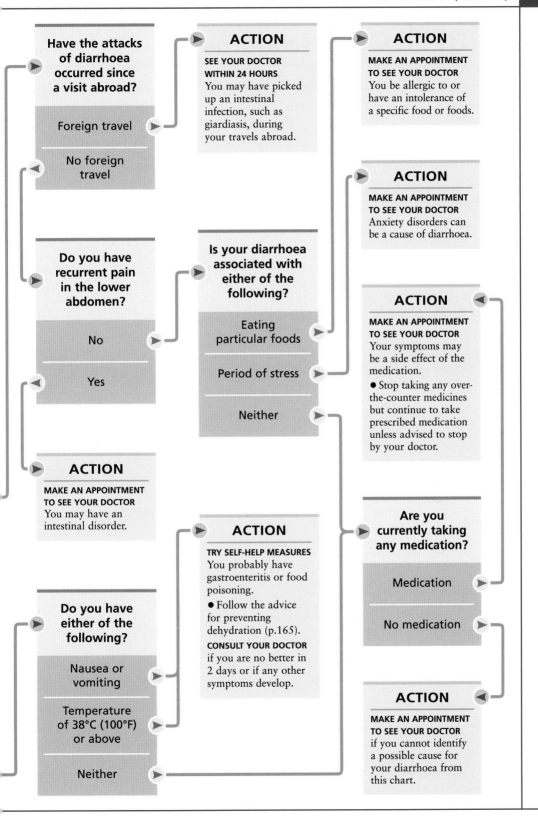

Have the attacks of diarrhoea occurred since a visit abroad?

Foreign travel

No foreign travel

ACTION

SEE YOUR DOCTOR WITHIN 24 HOURS
You may have picked up an intestinal infection, such as giardiasis, during your travels abroad.

ACTION

MAKE AN APPOINTMENT TO SEE YOUR DOCTOR
You be allergic to or have an intolerance of a specific food or foods.

ACTION

MAKE AN APPOINTMENT TO SEE YOUR DOCTOR
Anxiety disorders can be a cause of diarrhoea.

Do you have recurrent pain in the lower abdomen?

No

Yes

Is your diarrhoea associated with either of the following?

Eating particular foods

Period of stress

Neither

ACTION

MAKE AN APPOINTMENT TO SEE YOUR DOCTOR
Your symptoms may be a side effect of the medication.
● Stop taking any over-the-counter medicines but continue to take prescribed medication unless advised to stop by your doctor.

ACTION

MAKE AN APPOINTMENT TO SEE YOUR DOCTOR
You may have an intestinal disorder.

ACTION

TRY SELF-HELP MEASURES
You probably have gastroenteritis or food poisoning.
● Follow the advice for preventing dehydration (p.165).
CONSULT YOUR DOCTOR if you are no better in 2 days or if any other symptoms develop.

Are you currently taking any medication?

Medication

No medication

Do you have either of the following?

Nausea or vomiting

Temperature of 38°C (100°F) or above

Neither

ACTION

MAKE AN APPOINTMENT TO SEE YOUR DOCTOR
if you cannot identify a possible cause for your diarrhoea from this chart.

Diarrhoea (children)

◀ **For adults and children over 12, see p.128**
Diarrhoea is the passage of loose or watery faeces
more often than normal. Breast-fed babies may pass
loose faeces several times a day, and this is normal.
If your child has diarrhoea, he or she should drink
plenty of clear fluids to avoid dehydration. If
symptoms do not improve, consult your doctor.

Danger signs
Call an ambulance if your
child also has any of
the following symptoms:
● Abnormal drowsiness.
● Severe abdominal pain or
abdominal pain that lasts
for 4 hours or more.
● No urine passed during
the day for 3 hours (if
under 1 year) or 6 hours
(in an older child).
● Refusal to drink or feed
(in babies) for over 6 hours.
● Blood in the faeces.

START

How long has your child had diarrhoea?
- Less than 3 days
- 3 days or more

Does your child have any of the following?
- Abdominal pain
- Temperature of 38°C (100°F) or above
- Vomiting
- None of the above

ACTION
CALL YOUR DOCTOR NOW if your child is under 6
months. He or she may have gastroenteritis.
CONSULT YOUR DOCTOR if your child is over 6
months and not better within 24 hours or if
any other symptoms develop.
● Follow the advice for preventing dehydration (p.165).

ACTION
MAKE AN APPOINTMENT TO SEE YOUR DOCTOR
Persistent constipation can lead to faeces trickling from the anus, which may be mistaken for diarrhoea.

Is your child currently taking any medication?
- Medication
- No medication

Is your child gaining weight and growing normally (see growth charts, p.71)?
- Yes
- No

Was your child constipated before the onset of diarrhoea?
- Constipated
- Not constipated

What is the appearance of the faeces?
- Uniformly runny
- Contains pieces of food

ACTION

SEE YOUR DOCTOR WITHIN 24 HOURS
Your child's symptoms may be a side effect of the drug.
● Stop giving any over-the-counter medicines but continue to give prescribed medication unless advised to stop by your doctor.

How old is your child?

Under 12 months

12 months to 3 years

Over 3 years

ACTION

TRY SELF-HELP MEASURES
Young children often fail to chew and digest food properly, which can lead to so-called "toddler's diarrhoea".
● Follow the advice for preventing dehydration (p.165).
CONSULT YOUR DOCTOR
if symptoms persist or if your child develops other symptoms.

ACTION

MAKE AN APPOINTMENT TO SEE YOUR DOCTOR
It is possible that your child has a condition affecting the digestive tract, such as food intolerance or coeliac disease (gluten allergy).

Was your baby given any of the following before the onset of diarrhoea?

Unfamiliar foods

Sugary foods or sweetened drinks

Neither

ACTION

SEE YOUR DOCTOR WITHIN 24 HOURS
if you cannot identify a possible cause for your child's diarrhoea from this chart.

Is your child experiencing unusual stress, anxiety, or excitement?

Stress or anxiety

Excitement

Neither

ACTION

SEE YOUR DOCTOR WITHIN 24 HOURS
if you cannot identify a possible cause for your child's diarrhoea from this chart.

ACTION

TRY SELF-HELP MEASURES
Foods that are new to your baby may cause digestive upsets.
● Withhold the food that seems to be causing the trouble for at least 1 week.
CONSULT YOUR DOCTOR
if your baby is no better in 24 hours or if he or she develops other symptoms.

ACTION

TRY SELF-HELP MEASURES
Sugar in food and drink can cause diarrhoea in babies.
● Avoid giving your baby sweetened foods and drinks.
CONSULT YOUR DOCTOR
if your baby is no better in 24 hours or if he or she develops other symptoms.

ACTION

TRY SELF-HELP MEASURES
Psychological stress or unusual excitement can cause diarrhoea in children. The symptoms will normally stop as soon as the cause has disappeared.
CONSULT YOUR DOCTOR
if there is a long-term cause of anxiety in your child's life or if he or she develops other symptoms.

Constipation

Some people have a bowel movement once or twice a day; others do so less frequently. If you have fewer bowel movements than is usual for you or if your faeces are small and hard, you are constipated. The cause is often a lack of fluid or fibre-rich foods in the diet. If constipation occurs suddenly or persists despite a change in your diet, consult your doctor.

! Blood in the faeces

Blood can appear in the faeces as red streaks or in larger amounts. It can also make the stools look black. Small amounts of blood in the faeces are usually caused by minor anal problems, such as haemorrhoids, but you should always consult your doctor if you notice blood in the faeces because it is vital that other causes, such as colorectal cancer, are excluded.

START

How long have you suffered from constipation?

For a few weeks or less

For several months or years

Does either of the following apply?

You regularly ignore the urge to defeacate

You regularly use stimulant laxatives

Neither

Do you have pain in your rectum or anus when you defaecate?

Pain

No pain

Do you have intermittent bouts of cramping pain in the lower abdomen?

Pain

No pain

ACTION

MAKE AN APPOINTMENT TO SEE YOUR DOCTOR
Pain on defaecation can cause or worsen constipation. You may have haemorrhoids or anal fissure (a tear in the lining of the anus).

ACTION

TRY SELF-HELP MEASURES
Your bowel reflexes may have become sluggish as a result of being ignored.
● Include more fibre-rich foods in your diet.
● Increase your daily fluid intake.
CONSULT YOUR DOCTOR
if your symptoms have not improved within 2 weeks.

ACTION

MAKE AN APPOINTMENT TO SEE YOUR DOCTOR
Regular use of stimulant laxatives, such as senna, can seriously disrupt the normal functioning of the bowels.

ACTION

TRY SELF-HELP MEASURES
Your constipation is probably due to a lack of fibre or fluid in your diet and possibly to lack of exercise.
● Include more fibre-rich foods in your diet.
● Avoid eating too much processed food.
● Increase your daily fluid intake.
● Do not ignore the urge to defaecate.
CONSULT YOUR DOCTOR
if your symptoms have not improved within 2 weeks.

ACTION

**MAKE AN APPOINTMENT
TO SEE YOUR DOCTOR**
Irritable bowel
syndrome is a possible
cause, especially if
your constipation
alternates with bouts
of diarrhoea. However,
other causes, such as
cancer of the colon,
rectum, or anus, may
need to be ruled out.

Are you taking any medication?

Medication

No medication

ACTION

**MAKE AN APPOINTMENT
TO SEE YOUR DOCTOR**
Your symptoms may
be a side effect of the
medication.
● Stop taking any over-
the-counter medicines
but continue to take
prescribed medication
unless advised to stop
by your doctor.

Do you have any of the following?

Tiredness

Increased dryness
or roughness
of the skin

Feeling the cold
more than you
used to

Unexplained
weight gain

Generalized
hair thinning

None of
the above

Do any of the following apply?

You are
pregnant

You have been
drinking less fluid
than usual

You have changed
your diet

None of
the above

ACTION

TRY SELF-HELP MEASURES
Constipation is quite
common in pregnancy.
● Include more fibre-
rich foods in your diet.
● Avoid eating too
much processed food.
● Increase your daily
fluid intake, but avoid
caffeine and alcohol.
● Do not ignore the
urge to defaecate.
CONSULT YOUR DOCTOR
if your symptoms have
not improved within
2 weeks.

ACTION

TRY SELF-HELP MEASURES
Lack of fluid in the
bowel as a result of an
inadequate fluid intake
or excessive fluid loss
can cause constipation.
● Drink plenty of
fluids, especially if the
weather is hot.
CONSULT YOUR DOCTOR
if your symptoms have
not improved within
2 weeks.

ACTION

**MAKE AN APPOINTMENT
TO SEE YOUR DOCTOR**
Hypothyroidism
(underactivity of the
thyroid gland, which
causes many body
functions to slow
down) is a possibility.

ACTION

**MAKE AN APPOINTMENT
TO SEE YOUR DOCTOR**
if you cannot identify
a possible cause for
your constipation from
this chart.

ACTION

TRY SELF-HELP MEASURES
A change in your
regular diet, especially
when travelling, can
make you constipated.
● Include more fibre-
rich foods in your diet.
● Avoid eating too
much processed food.
● Increase your daily
fluid intake.
● Do not ignore the
urge to defaecate.
CONSULT YOUR DOCTOR
if your symptoms have
not improved within
2 weeks.

Chest pain

Pain in the chest, or any discomfort felt in the front or back of the ribcage, is most often due to minor disorders such as muscle strain or indigestion. However, you should call an ambulance if you have a crushing pain in the centre or left side of your chest, if you are also short of breath or feel faint, or if the pain is unlike any pain you have had before.

START

What kind of pain are you experiencing?

Crushing

Spreading from the centre of the chest to the neck, arms, or jaw

Neither of the above

Does the pain subside after you rest for a few minutes?

Pain subsides

Pain persists

ACTION

! **CALL AN AMBULANCE**
■ You may be having a heart attack.
● While waiting, chew half an aspirin, unless you are allergic to it.

Are you short of breath?

Short of breath

Not short of breath

ACTION

CALL YOUR DOCTOR NOW
Recurrent chest pain could be an indication of angina, especially if pain in the chest occurs with exertion and disappears with rest.

Have you had this pain before?

Previous episodes of this kind of pain

Never before

ACTION

! **CALL AN AMBULANCE**
■ You may have a blood clot in the lung.

Do any of the following apply?

You have recently had surgery

You have recently been immobile due to injury or illness

You have had a baby within the past 2 weeks

None of the above

Is pain related to breathing?

Related to breathing

Not related to breathing

ACTION

! **CALL AN AMBULANCE**
■ You may be having a heart attack.
● While waiting, chew half an aspirin, unless you are allergic to it.

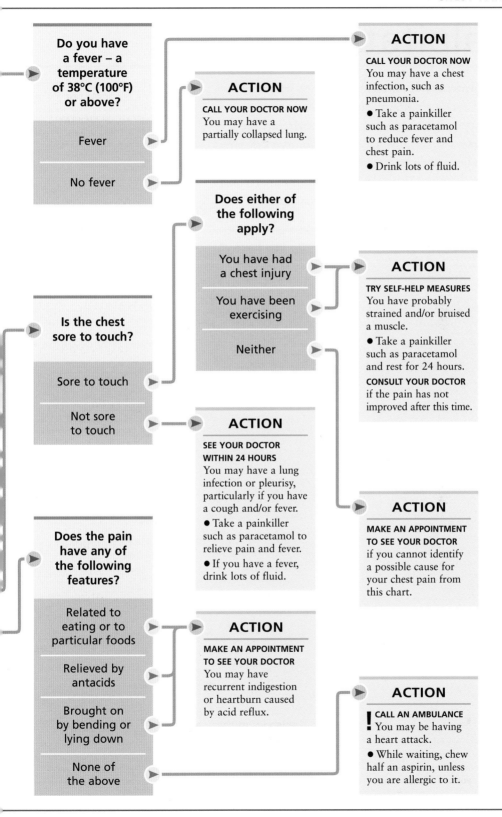

Do you have a fever – a temperature of 38°C (100°F) or above?

Fever

No fever

ACTION

CALL YOUR DOCTOR NOW
You may have a chest infection, such as pneumonia.
● Take a painkiller such as paracetamol to reduce fever and chest pain.
● Drink lots of fluid.

ACTION

CALL YOUR DOCTOR NOW
You may have a partially collapsed lung.

Does either of the following apply?

You have had a chest injury

You have been exercising

Neither

ACTION

TRY SELF-HELP MEASURES
You have probably strained and/or bruised a muscle.
● Take a painkiller such as paracetamol and rest for 24 hours.
CONSULT YOUR DOCTOR
if the pain has not improved after this time.

Is the chest sore to touch?

Sore to touch

Not sore to touch

ACTION

SEE YOUR DOCTOR
WITHIN 24 HOURS
You may have a lung infection or pleurisy, particularly if you have a cough and/or fever.
● Take a painkiller such as paracetamol to relieve pain and fever.
● If you have a fever, drink lots of fluid.

ACTION

MAKE AN APPOINTMENT TO SEE YOUR DOCTOR
if you cannot identify a possible cause for your chest pain from this chart.

Does the pain have any of the following features?

Related to eating or to particular foods

Relieved by antacids

Brought on by bending or lying down

None of the above

ACTION

MAKE AN APPOINTMENT TO SEE YOUR DOCTOR
You may have recurrent indigestion or heartburn caused by acid reflux.

ACTION

! CALL AN AMBULANCE
You may be having a heart attack.
● While waiting, chew half an aspirin, unless you are allergic to it.

Palpitations

An awareness of abnormally fast or irregular heartbeats, or palpitations, is often caused by anxiety or by stimulants, such as caffeine and nicotine. Palpitations may also occur as a side effect of medication or because of a heart disorder. Call your doctor immediately if palpitations are frequent or persistent or if you have other symptoms.

START

Do you have any of the following?

- Shortness of breath
- Chest discomfort
- Feeling faint or passing out
- None of the above

ACTION

! **CALL AN AMBULANCE**
You may have a serious arrhythmia (abnormal heart rate or rhythm) due to an underlying heart disorder.

ACTION

SEE YOUR DOCTOR WITHIN 24 HOURS
Your symptoms may be a side effect of the medication.

● Stop taking any over-the-counter medicines but continue to take prescribed medication unless advised to stop by your doctor.

Do you have any of the following?

- Weight loss with increased appetite
- Feeling on edge
- Increased sweating
- Bulging eyes
- None of the above

Do any of the following apply?

- You have been drinking a lot of coffee, tea, or cola
- You have been smoking more than usual
- You are taking medications
- None of the above

ACTION

MAKE AN APPOINTMENT TO SEE YOUR DOCTOR
You may have hyperthyroidism (an overactive thyroid gland) or be suffering from anxiety.

ACTION

TRY SELF-HELP MEASURES
These symptoms may be due to anxiety.

● Try some relaxation exercises (p.169).

CONSULT YOUR DOCTOR
if your symptoms continue for 2 days.

ACTION

TRY SELF-HELP MEASURES
● Avoid caffeine and nicotine as these can disturb your heart rhythm.

CONSULT YOUR DOCTOR
if your symptoms continue for 2 days.

Have you been feeling tense or stressed?

- Feeling under stress
- No increase in stress

ACTION

MAKE AN APPOINTMENT TO SEE YOUR DOCTOR
if you cannot identify a possible cause for your palpitations from this chart.

Poor bladder control

If passing urine is painful, see p.138 ▶
Inability to control the passage of urine may result in leakage of urine or difficulty urinating. These symptoms may be due to a bladder, nerve, or muscle disorder. In men, an enlarged prostate gland is a common cause. Urinary tract infections can also cause leakage of urine, especially in elderly people.

❗ Inability to pass urine

Inability to pass urine, even though the bladder is full, is a serious symptom. It may be the result of an obstruction or damage to nerves that supply the bladder, or it may be a side effect of certain drugs. You should telephone your doctor immediately.

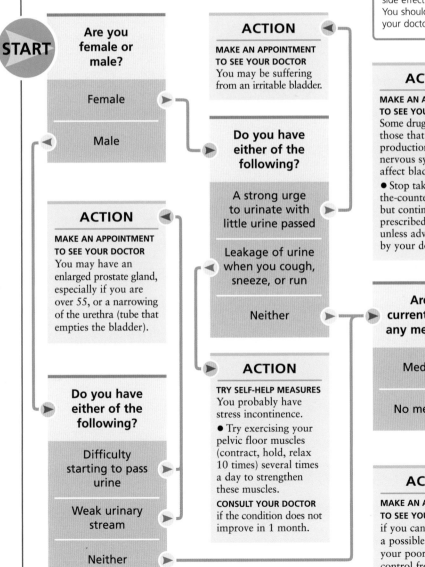

START

Are you female or male?

Female ▶

Male ◀

ACTION

MAKE AN APPOINTMENT TO SEE YOUR DOCTOR
You may be suffering from an irritable bladder.

Do you have either of the following?

A strong urge to urinate with little urine passed ▶

Leakage of urine when you cough, sneeze, or run ◀

Neither ▶

ACTION

MAKE AN APPOINTMENT TO SEE YOUR DOCTOR
Some drugs, particularly those that act on urine production or on the nervous system, can affect bladder control.
● Stop taking any over-the-counter medicines but continue to take prescribed medication unless advised to stop by your doctor.

Are you currently taking any medication?

Medication ▶

No medication ▶

ACTION

MAKE AN APPOINTMENT TO SEE YOUR DOCTOR
You may have an enlarged prostate gland, especially if you are over 55, or a narrowing of the urethra (tube that empties the bladder).

Do you have either of the following?

Difficulty starting to pass urine ▶

Weak urinary stream ▶

Neither ▶

ACTION

TRY SELF-HELP MEASURES
You probably have stress incontinence.
● Try exercising your pelvic floor muscles (contract, hold, relax 10 times) several times a day to strengthen these muscles.

CONSULT YOUR DOCTOR if the condition does not improve in 1 month.

ACTION

MAKE AN APPOINTMENT TO SEE YOUR DOCTOR
if you cannot identify a possible cause for your poor bladder control from this chart.

Painful urination

Pain or discomfort while passing urine is usually caused by inflammation of the urinary tract, often due to infection. Frequent painless urination can be due to diabetes or kidney problems and should be investigated by your doctor. Discoloured urine can accompany this type of pain but may not indicate disease (see Checking the appearance of urine, right).

Checking the appearance of urine

The appearance of urine varies considerably. For example, urine is often darker in the morning than later in the day. Some drugs and foods may also cause a temporary colour change in the urine. Beetroot, for example, may turn the urine red. A change in your urine can indicate a disorder. Very dark urine may be a sign of liver disease, such as acute hepatitis, while red or cloudy urine may be due to bleeding or an infection in the kidney or bladder.

● If you are not sure about the cause of a change in the appearance of your urine, consult your doctor.

START

Do you have either of the following?

Pain in the back just above the waist

A temperature of 38°C (100°F) or above

Neither

ACTION

CALL YOUR DOCTOR NOW
You may have pyelonephritis (infection of the kidneys).

● Take a painkiller such as paracetamol.

Have you felt the need to pass urine more frequently than usual?

Increased frequency

No increased frequency

Do you have any of the following?

Lower abdominal pain

Blood in the urine

Cloudy urine

None of the above

ACTION

SEE YOUR DOCTOR WITHIN 24 HOURS
You may have cystitis.

● Take a painkiller such as paracetamol.
● Drink 500 ml (1 pt) of fluid every hour for 4 hours.
● Drinking cranberry juice may help relieve the burning sensation.

Are you female or male?

Female

Male

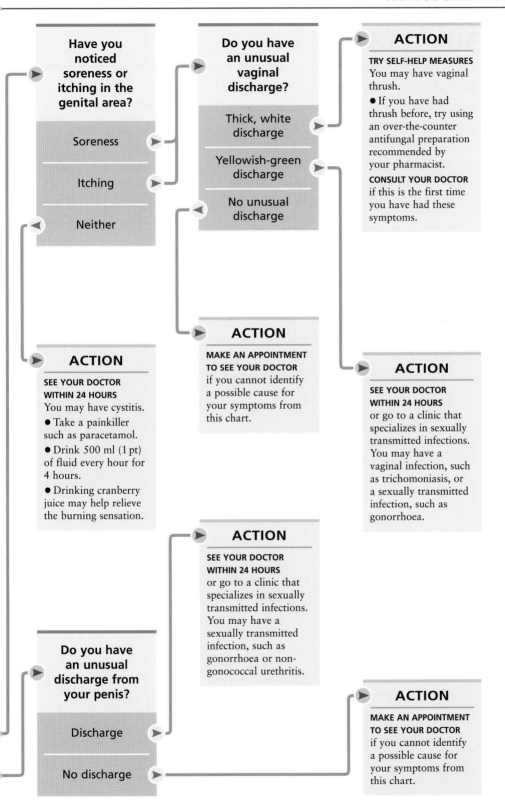

Have you noticed soreness or itching in the genital area?

Soreness

Itching

Neither

Do you have an unusual vaginal discharge?

Thick, white discharge

Yellowish-green discharge

No unusual discharge

ACTION

TRY SELF-HELP MEASURES
You may have vaginal thrush.

● If you have had thrush before, try using an over-the-counter antifungal preparation recommended by your pharmacist.

CONSULT YOUR DOCTOR
if this is the first time you have had these symptoms.

ACTION

SEE YOUR DOCTOR WITHIN 24 HOURS
You may have cystitis.

● Take a painkiller such as paracetamol.

● Drink 500 ml (1 pt) of fluid every hour for 4 hours.

● Drinking cranberry juice may help relieve the burning sensation.

ACTION

MAKE AN APPOINTMENT TO SEE YOUR DOCTOR
if you cannot identify a possible cause for your symptoms from this chart.

ACTION

SEE YOUR DOCTOR WITHIN 24 HOURS
or go to a clinic that specializes in sexually transmitted infections. You may have a vaginal infection, such as trichomoniasis, or a sexually transmitted infection, such as gonorrhoea.

ACTION

SEE YOUR DOCTOR WITHIN 24 HOURS
or go to a clinic that specializes in sexually transmitted infections. You may have a sexually transmitted infection, such as gonorrhoea or non-gonococcal urethritis.

Do you have an unusual discharge from your penis?

Discharge

No discharge

ACTION

MAKE AN APPOINTMENT TO SEE YOUR DOCTOR
if you cannot identify a possible cause for your symptoms from this chart.

Back pain

Mild back pain is usually caused by poor posture, sudden movement, or lifting heavy objects, all of which may strain the back. Back pain is also common in pregnancy. Persistent or severe back pain may be the result of a more serious problem. You should consult your doctor if pain is severe or does not start to improve after 48 hours.

Danger signs

Call an ambulance if you have back pain that is associated with one of the following symptoms:
- Difficulty in controlling your bladder.
- Difficulty in controlling your bowels.

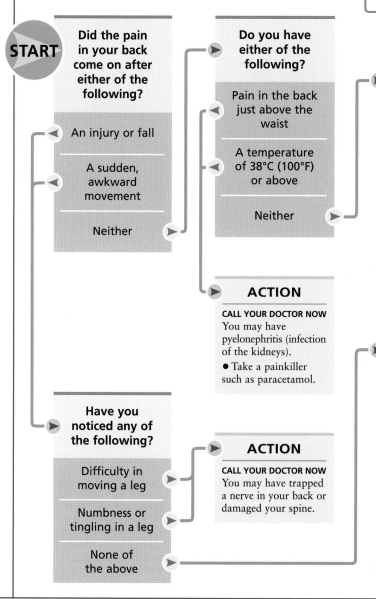

START

Did the pain in your back come on after either of the following?

An injury or fall

A sudden, awkward movement

Neither

Do you have either of the following?

Pain in the back just above the waist

A temperature of 38°C (100°F) or above

Neither

Did the pain occur after any of the following?

Lifting a heavy weight

A fit of coughing

Strenuous or unaccustomed physical activity

None of the above

ACTION

CALL YOUR DOCTOR NOW
You may have pyelonephritis (infection of the kidneys).
- Take a painkiller such as paracetamol.

Have you noticed any of the following?

Difficulty in moving a leg

Numbness or tingling in a leg

None of the above

ACTION

CALL YOUR DOCTOR NOW
You may have trapped a nerve in your back or damaged your spine.

ACTION

TRY SELF-HELP MEASURES
You have probably strained a back muscle and/or bruised your back by overstretching a muscle.
- Take a painkiller such as paracetamol and rest.
- A covered hot-water bottle or a heat pad placed against your back may give you additional pain relief.

CONSULT YOUR DOCTOR
if you are no better within 24 hours.

Does either of the following apply?

Pain makes any movement difficult

Pain shoots from the spine down the back of the leg

Neither

ACTION

SEE YOUR DOCTOR WITHIN 24 HOURS
You may have fractured a vertebra as a result of osteoporosis or have sciatica caused by a slipped disc.

ACTION

MAKE AN APPOINTMENT TO SEE YOUR DOCTOR
You may have osteoarthritis.

ACTION

MAKE AN APPOINTMENT TO SEE YOUR DOCTOR
You may have ankylosing spondylitis (a form of arthritis affecting the back of the pelvis and the vertebrae of the spine), especially if you are male.

How old are you?

45 or over

Under 45

ACTION

TRY SELF-HELP MEASURES
You have probably strained some of the muscles or sprained some of the ligaments in your back.
● Take a painkiller such as paracetamol.
● Place a covered hot-water bottle or a heat pad against your back to ease the pain.
CONSULT YOUR DOCTOR
if you do not feel any better in 2 or 3 days or if any other symptoms develop.

ACTION

SEE YOUR DOCTOR WITHIN 24 HOURS
You may have fractured a vertebra as a result of osteoporosis.

ACTION

CALL YOUR DOCTOR OR MIDWIFE NOW
New back pain or a worsening of existing back pain may indicate the start of labour.

Are you in the last 3 months of pregnancy?

Pregnant

Not pregnant

Have you been suffering from increasing pain and stiffness over several months?

Yes

No

Does either of the following apply?

You are over 60

You have recently been immobile due to illness or injury

Neither

ACTION

MAKE AN APPOINTMENT TO SEE YOUR DOCTOR
if you cannot identify a possible cause for your back pain from this chart.

Neck pain or stiffness

Pain and/or stiffness in the neck is usually due to a minor problem, such as muscle strain or ligament sprain, that does not require treatment. However, if the pain occurs with fever, meningitis is a possibility. Neck pain or stiffness becomes more common as a person gets older and may then be due to a disorder of the bones and joints of the neck.

Danger signs

Call an ambulance if you have neck pain associated with any of the following:
- Difficulty in controlling your bladder.
- Difficulty in controlling your bowels.
- Severe headache.
- Drowsiness or confusion.
- Dislike of bright light.

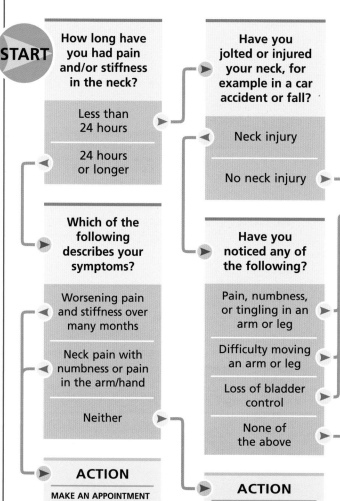

START

How long have you had pain and/or stiffness in the neck?

Less than 24 hours

24 hours or longer

Have you jolted or injured your neck, for example in a car accident or fall?

Neck injury

No neck injury

Which of the following describes your symptoms?

Worsening pain and stiffness over many months

Neck pain with numbness or pain in the arm/hand

Neither

Have you noticed any of the following?

Pain, numbness, or tingling in an arm or leg

Difficulty moving an arm or leg

Loss of bladder control

None of the above

ACTION

! CALL AN AMBULANCE You may have damaged your spine.
- Follow the first-aid advice for spinal injuries (p.46).

ACTION

TRY SELF-HELP MEASURES Your neck is probably strained and/or bruised from overstretching a muscle.
- Take a painkiller such as paracetamol and rest lying down.
- A heat pad or covered hot-water bottle placed against your neck may give additional pain relief.

CONSULT YOUR DOCTOR if you are no better in 24 hours.

ACTION

MAKE AN APPOINTMENT TO SEE YOUR DOCTOR You may have osteoarthritis of the upper spine, especially if you are over the age of 45.

ACTION

MAKE AN APPOINTMENT TO SEE YOUR DOCTOR if you cannot identify a possible cause for your neck pain or stiffness from this chart.

Do you have any of the following?

Temperature of 38°C (100°F) or above

Severe headache

Drowsiness or confusion

Dislike of bright light

Nausea or vomiting

None of the above

Does either of the following apply?

Pain is severe enough to prevent movement

Pain shoots down one arm from the neck

Neither

ACTION

SEE YOUR DOCTOR WITHIN 24 HOURS Your neck pain may be due to pressure on a nerve as a result of a slipped disc or osteoarthritis of the upper spine.

ACTION

TRY SELF-HELP MEASURES You may have neck strain caused by overstretching a muscle.
● Rest your neck as much as possible by lying down.
● Take a nonsteroidal anti-inflammatory drug, such as ibuprofen, to ease the pain.
● Keeping your neck warm with a heat pad or covered hot-water bottle may also help.
CONSULT YOUR DOCTOR if you are no better in 3 days.

ACTION

! CALL AN AMBULANCE You may have meningitis (infection inflaming membranes around the brain).

Can you feel any tenderness or swelling at the sides or the back of the neck?

Yes

No

ACTION

GO TO ANOTHER CHART Lumps and swellings, p.80

Did either of the following apply in the 24 hours before the onset of pain?

You exercised unusually strenuously

You sat or slept in an awkward position

Neither

ACTION

MAKE AN APPOINTMENT TO SEE YOUR DOCTOR if you cannot identify a possible cause for your neck pain or stiffness from this chart.

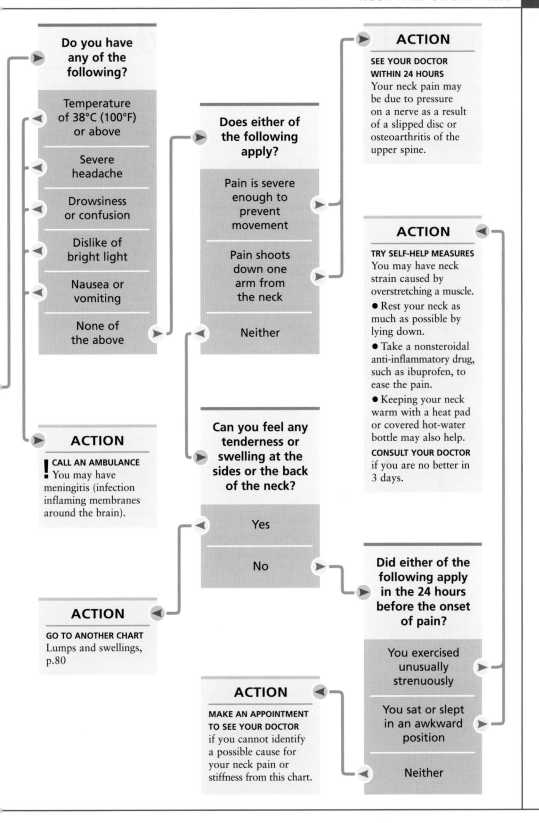

Painful arm or hand

If you have painful joints, see p.146 ▶

Pain in the arm or hand is often caused by injury or a problem in the neck or shoulder. Rarely, pain in the arm is due to a heart attack or a serious neck disorder. Consult your doctor if the pain is severe, recurrent, or persistent.

ACTION

MAKE AN APPOINTMENT TO SEE YOUR DOCTOR
You may have repetitive strain injury.
● Take a painkiller such as paracetamol.

START

Did the pain start during or soon after either of the following?

- An injury or fall
- Repetitive arm or hand movements
- Neither

Is the pain associated with any of the following?

- Chest tightness
- Shortness of breath
- Nausea, sweating, or feeling faint
- None of the above

ACTION

❗ CALL AN AMBULANCE
You may be having a heart attack.
● While waiting, chew half an aspirin, unless you are allergic to it.

ACTION

MAKE AN APPOINTMENT TO SEE YOUR DOCTOR
You may have inflammation of a tendon or polymyalgia, in which muscles become inflamed, particularly if you are over 60 years old.

ACTION

CALL YOUR DOCTOR NOW
if you are in severe pain. You may have either fractured a bone or damaged a muscle.
● Follow the first-aid advice for a broken arm (p.44).
TRY SELF-HELP MEASURES
if not in severe pain.
● Follow the first-aid advice for sprains and strains (p.47).

What are the features of the pain?

- Localized in upper arm or shoulder
- Extends from the wrist into the palm and lower arm
- Shoots down the length of the arm
- None of the above

ACTION

SEE YOUR DOCTOR WITHIN 24 HOURS
You may have a pinched nerve in your neck.

ACTION

MAKE AN APPOINTMENT TO SEE YOUR DOCTOR
You may have a trapped nerve in the wrist (carpal tunnel syndrome).

ACTION

MAKE AN APPOINTMENT TO SEE YOUR DOCTOR
if you cannot identify a possible cause for your painful arm or hand from this chart.

Painful leg

If you have painful joints, see p.146 ▶
Leg pain due to a pulled muscle or torn ligament
usually goes away without treatment. Pain may
also result from a problem in the lower back or
in the blood vessels in the leg. If your leg is also
swollen, hot, or red, see your doctor at once.

ACTION

**SEE YOUR DOCTOR
WITHIN 24 HOURS**
Your symptoms may
be caused by cellulitis
(infection of the skin
and underlying
tissue) or superficial
thrombophlebitis
(inflamed surface vein).

START

Did the pain
start during or
soon after
either of the
following?

An injury or fall

Unaccustomed
exercise

Neither

ACTION

TRY SELF-HELP MEASURES
You may have strained
a muscle.
● Follow the first-aid
advice for sprains and
strains (p.47).

What are the
features of
the pain?

Affects a small
area that is also
red and hot

Sudden tightening
of calf muscles

Constant pain in
the calf, which
may be swollen

Shooting pain
down the back
of the leg

Heavy,
aching legs

None of
the above

ACTION

**MAKE AN APPOINTMENT
TO SEE YOUR DOCTOR**
You may have muscle
cramp, but, if the pain
occurs with exercise
and disappears with
rest, you may have
claudication due to
narrowing of the blood
vessels in the leg.

ACTION

**MAKE AN APPOINTMENT
TO SEE YOUR DOCTOR**
Varicose veins are a
possible cause.

Does sitting
down with your
feet up relieve
the pain?

Yes

No

ACTION

CALL YOUR DOCTOR NOW
if you are in severe
pain. You may have
either fractured a bone
or damaged a muscle.
● Follow the first-aid
advice for a broken
leg (p.45).
TRY SELF-HELP MEASURES
if not in severe pain.
● Follow the first-aid
advice for sprains and
strains (p.47).

ACTION

CALL YOUR DOCTOR NOW
You may have deep
vein thrombosis
(blood clot in a vein
in your leg).

ACTION

**MAKE AN APPOINTMENT
TO SEE YOUR DOCTOR**
You may have sciatica.

ACTION

**MAKE AN APPOINTMENT
TO SEE YOUR DOCTOR**
if you cannot identify
a possible cause for
your painful leg from
this chart.

Painful joints

If your ankle is swollen painlessly, see p.148 ▶
Pain in a joint may be caused by injury or strain
and often disappears without a cause being found.
Gout or a joint infection can cause a joint to
become red, hot, and swollen. Joint pain may also
be due to arthritis or a reaction to an infection.
Consult your doctor if pain is severe or persistent.

How many joints are affected?

One joint

More than one

START

Have you injured the joint?

Injury

No injury

Do you have either of the following?

Hot joint(s)

Red joint(s)

Neither

ACTION

SEE YOUR DOCTOR WITHIN 24 HOURS
You may have septic
arthritis (infected joint)
or gout.
● Rest the painful joint.
● Take ibuprofen at the
recommended intervals.
● Drink lots of fluid.

Does either of the following apply?

You cannot move the joint

The joint appears misshapen or swollen

Neither

ACTION

CALL YOUR DOCTOR NOW
You may have fractured
a bone, strained or
torn a muscle, or torn
a ligament.
● Follow the first-aid
advice for a broken arm
or leg (pp.44–45).

Does moving the joint affect the pain?

Considerably worsens it

Slightly worsens it or no change

ACTION

TRY SELF-HELP MEASURES
You have probably
strained a ligament
around the joint.
● Follow the first-aid
advice for sprains and
strains (p.47).
CONSULT YOUR DOCTOR
if the joint is no better
in 24 hours.

ACTION

MAKE AN APPOINTMENT TO SEE YOUR DOCTOR
You may have
osteoarthritis.
● Take a painkiller
such as paracetamol.
● Put a covered hot-
water bottle or heat
pad on the joint.

Did the pain come on gradually over months or years?

Yes

No

Have you recently had either of the following?

- An infection with a rash
- An infection without a rash
- Neither

ACTION

SEE YOUR DOCTOR WITHIN 24 HOURS
Certain bacterial infections of the intestines and genital tract can lead to reactive arthritis (short-term inflammation of the joint).

ACTION

SEE YOUR DOCTOR WITHIN 24 HOURS
Some viral illnesses, such as rubella (German measles), can cause joint pain, but an infection such as Lyme disease could be the cause of joint pains if you have been bitten by a tick.

ACTION

SEE YOUR DOCTOR WITHIN 24 HOURS
You may have rheumatoid arthritis.
- Take a painkiller such as ibuprofen.

ACTION

MAKE AN APPOINTMENT TO SEE YOUR DOCTOR
You may have a frozen shoulder.
- Take a painkiller such as paracetamol to ease the pain.
- Rest your shoulder.

Is the problem in a child aged under 12?

- Under 12
- 12 or over

Which joint or joints are affected?

- Shoulder
- Hip
- Neck
- Other joint(s)

ACTION

TRY SELF-HELP MEASURES
Your symptoms are probably a result of overuse, although recent viral illness may also be the cause.
- Rest the painful joint(s).
- Take a painkiller such as paracetamol to ease the pain.

CONSULT YOUR DOCTOR
if your condition is no better in 2 days.

ACTION

SEE YOUR DOCTOR WITHIN 24 HOURS
Most childhood hip problems are not serious, but some need prompt treatment to prevent lasting damage being done to the joint.

ACTION

GO TO ANOTHER CHART
Neck pain or stiffness, p.142

ACTION

MAKE AN APPOINTMENT TO SEE YOUR DOCTOR
if you cannot identify a possible cause for your painful joints from this chart.

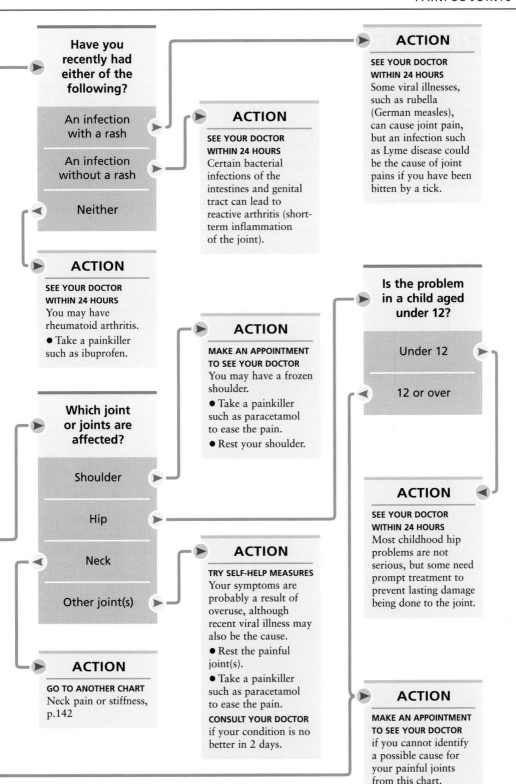

Swollen ankles

◄ If you have a painful swollen ankle, see p.146

Slight, painless swelling of the ankles is most often caused by fluid accumulating in the tissues after long periods of sitting or standing still, but it may be due to heart, liver, or kidney disorders. It is common in pregnancy. If swelling persists or if you have other symptoms, consult your doctor.

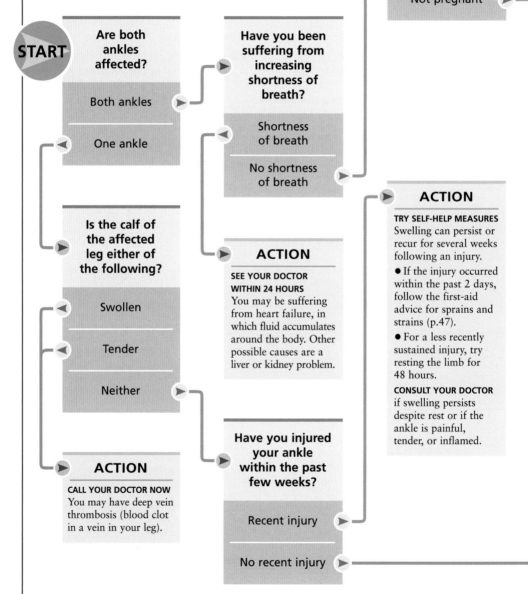

START

Are both ankles affected?

Both ankles

One ankle

Have you been suffering from increasing shortness of breath?

Shortness of breath

No shortness of breath

Is the calf of the affected leg either of the following?

Swollen

Tender

Neither

ACTION

SEE YOUR DOCTOR WITHIN 24 HOURS
You may be suffering from heart failure, in which fluid accumulates around the body. Other possible causes are a liver or kidney problem.

ACTION

CALL YOUR DOCTOR NOW
You may have deep vein thrombosis (blood clot in a vein in your leg).

Have you injured your ankle within the past few weeks?

Recent injury

No recent injury

Are you pregnant?

Pregnant

Not pregnant

ACTION

TRY SELF-HELP MEASURES
Swelling can persist or recur for several weeks following an injury.

● If the injury occurred within the past 2 days, follow the first-aid advice for sprains and strains (p.47).

● For a less recently sustained injury, try resting the limb for 48 hours.

CONSULT YOUR DOCTOR
if swelling persists despite rest or if the ankle is painful, tender, or inflamed.

Does either of the following apply?

Your face or fingers are swollen

You have gained over 2 kg (4.5 lb) in the past week

Neither

ACTION

CALL YOUR DOCTOR OR MIDWIFE NOW
Retaining excessive amounts of fluid may be a symptom of pre-eclampsia, which, if severe, can be serious.

ACTION

TRY SELF-HELP MEASURES
Swollen ankles are common in pregnancy, particularly in the last 3 months.
- Avoid standing still for long periods.
- Put your feet up whenever possible.

CONSULT YOUR DOCTOR
if your face and/or fingers become swollen or if you start to put on weight rapidly.

Did your ankles become swollen during either of the following?

A long train, car, or coach trip

Aeroplane flight

Neither

ACTION

TRY SELF-HELP MEASURES
Hours of inactivity will lead to accumulation of fluid in the ankles and increases the risk of developing a blood clot.
- Clear excess fluid by taking a brisk walk.
- Avoid sitting or standing still for long periods.
- When seated, keep your legs raised.

ACTION

MAKE AN APPOINTMENT TO SEE YOUR DOCTOR
Your symptom may be a side effect of the drug.
- Stop taking any over-the-counter medicines but continue to take prescribed medication unless advised to stop by your doctor.

Are you currently taking any medication?

Medication

No medication

ACTION

TRY SELF-HELP MEASURES
You may have varicose veins, which can cause fluid to accumulate in the ankles.
- Avoid standing still for long periods.
- Walk as much as possible.
- When sitting down, try to keep your feet raised above hip level.
- Wear support tights.

CONSULT YOUR DOCTOR
if the swelling worsens or if other symptoms develop.

Do you have prominent veins in the leg or legs affected by swelling?

Prominent veins

No prominent veins

ACTION

MAKE AN APPOINTMENT TO SEE YOUR DOCTOR
if you cannot identify a possible cause for your swollen ankles from this chart.

Impotence

Occasional incidences of impotence, or failure to have or maintain an erection, are not uncommon. Difficulties are usually caused by factors such as stress, tiredness, anxiety, or alcohol. Physical causes are not common. If impotence occurs frequently, you should consult your doctor for advice. Safe and effective treatments for impotence are available.

Nonmedical advice

Treatment from a nonmedical source could result in the incorrect diagnosis being made or the wrong treatment given. It is important that you consult a doctor, who can rule out any medical cause of your erection problems, before having any form of treatment.

START

Are you interested in sex?

Yes

No

How often do you fail to achieve or maintain an erection?

Only occasionally

Frequently

ACTION

CONSULT YOUR DOCTOR if you are concerned about any problems with your sexual performance. Most men have occasional erection problems, most likely due to anxiety – for example at the beginning of a new sexual relationship – or due to factors such as tiredness or drinking too much alcohol.

ACTION

MAKE AN APPOINTMENT TO SEE YOUR DOCTOR Certain illnesses, such as diabetes, can lead to erection problems. Some drugs, including those prescribed for high blood pressure and antidepressants, can also have an effect on sexual performance.

Are you currently receiving treatment for an illness?

Treatment

No treatment

ACTION

MAKE AN APPOINTMENT TO SEE YOUR DOCTOR Lack of interest in sex is likely to reduce your ability to achieve an erection.

ACTION

MAKE AN APPOINTMENT TO SEE YOUR DOCTOR Anxiety about your sexual performance is the most likely explanation for your problem. A physical cause is unlikely.

Do you wake with an erection?

Sometimes

Never

ACTION

MAKE AN APPOINTMENT TO SEE YOUR DOCTOR if you cannot identify a possible cause for your erection problem from this chart.

Testes/scrotum problems

Check regularly for lumps or swellings in the testes, the sperm-producing organs, and the scrotum, the sac containing the testes (see Testes: self-examination, p.69). The cause may be minor, but there is a possibility of cancer of the testis, which is easily treated if diagnosed early. Painful swelling in the genital area requires immediate medical attention.

START

What is the nature of your symptoms?

- Pain and swelling
- Painless enlargement in or near testis
- Generalized painless swelling of the scrotum
- None of the above

Does the problem affect one or both testes?

- One
- Both

ACTION

! CALL AN AMBULANCE
You may have torsion, or twisting, of the testis, especially if the pain is severe, which can result in permanent damage if not treated promptly. A less serious possible cause is inflammation of the epididymis (sperm-carrying tube), especially if you also have a fever.

ACTION

CALL YOUR DOCTOR NOW
Internal damage to the testes is a possibility.

Have you had an injury in the genital area within the past 48 hours?

- Injury
- No injury

ACTION

MAKE AN APPOINTMENT TO SEE YOUR DOCTOR
You may have one of the following disorders of the scrotum: an accumulation of fluid, a hernia, or varicose veins. However, the slight possibility of cancer of the testis needs to be ruled out.

ACTION

SEE YOUR DOCTOR WITHIN 24 HOURS
You may have an infection of the testes or epididymides (sperm-carrying tubes). The cause could be a viral infection, such as mumps, or a sexually transmitted infection.

ACTION

MAKE AN APPOINTMENT TO SEE YOUR DOCTOR
You probably have a cyst in the epididymis (sperm-carrying tube in the scrotum). However, the slight possibility of cancer of the testis needs to be ruled out.

ACTION

MAKE AN APPOINTMENT TO SEE YOUR DOCTOR
if you cannot identify a possible cause for your testes or scrotum problem from this chart.

Penis problems

◀ If you are impotent, see p.150

Pain or soreness of the penis that is not related to injury is often due to infection in the urinary tract or of the skin of the penis. Inflammation may be caused by friction during sexual intercourse. You should consult your doctor if there is any change in the appearance of the skin of the penis.

Blood in the semen

Blood-streaked semen is usually caused by leakage from small blood vessels in the testes or epididymis. A single episode is unlikely to be a cause for concern, but, if it recurs, you should consult your doctor. It is also important to consult your doctor if you notice a blood-stained discharge that is not related to ejaculation or if you notice blood in your urine.

START

What is the problem?

- Painful or sore penis
- Discharge from penis
- Foreskin problem
- Change in appearance of erect penis
- None of the above

When does the pain occur?

- Only with an erection
- Only when passing urine
- At other times

ACTION

GO TO ANOTHER CHART
Painful urination, p.138

How is the foreskin affected?

- After retraction, cannot be replaced
- After childhood, cannot be fully retracted
- Balloons when passing urine
- None of the above

ACTION

❗ CALL AN AMBULANCE
Inability to replace a retracted foreskin (paraphimosis) can restrict the blood flow.

• While waiting, place an ice pack against the affected area.

ACTION

SEE YOUR DOCTOR
WITHIN 24 HOURS
or go to a clinic for sexually transmitted infections. You may have a sexually transmitted infection such as gonorrhoea.

ACTION

MAKE AN APPOINTMENT
TO SEE YOUR DOCTOR
You may have Peyronie's disease, which causes curvature of the erect penis.

ACTION

MAKE AN APPOINTMENT
TO SEE YOUR DOCTOR
An abnormally tight foreskin may cause these problems.

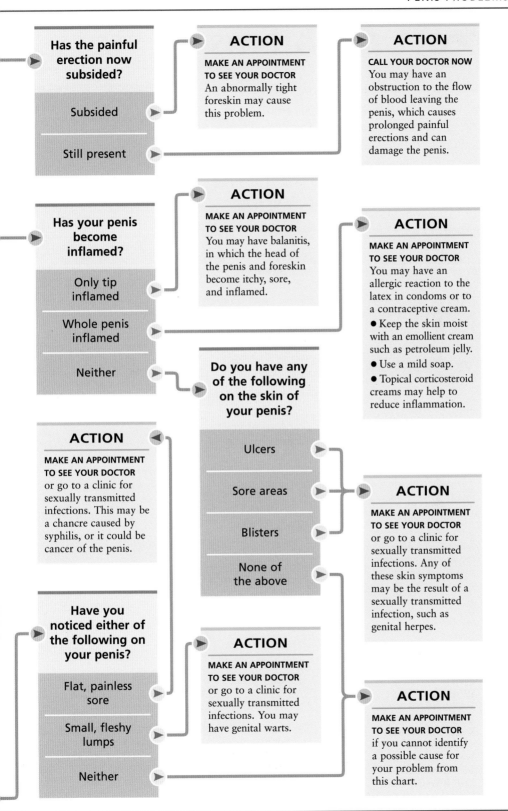

Has the painful erection now subsided?

Subsided ▶

Still present ▶

ACTION

MAKE AN APPOINTMENT TO SEE YOUR DOCTOR
An abnormally tight foreskin may cause this problem.

ACTION

CALL YOUR DOCTOR NOW
You may have an obstruction to the flow of blood leaving the penis, which causes prolonged painful erections and can damage the penis.

Has your penis become inflamed?

Only tip inflamed ▶

Whole penis inflamed ▶

Neither ▶

ACTION

MAKE AN APPOINTMENT TO SEE YOUR DOCTOR
You may have balanitis, in which the head of the penis and foreskin become itchy, sore, and inflamed.

ACTION

MAKE AN APPOINTMENT TO SEE YOUR DOCTOR
You may have an allergic reaction to the latex in condoms or to a contraceptive cream.
● Keep the skin moist with an emollient cream such as petroleum jelly.
● Use a mild soap.
● Topical corticosteroid creams may help to reduce inflammation.

Do you have any of the following on the skin of your penis?

Ulcers ▶

Sore areas ▶

Blisters ▶

None of the above ▶

ACTION

MAKE AN APPOINTMENT TO SEE YOUR DOCTOR
or go to a clinic for sexually transmitted infections. This may be a chancre caused by syphilis, or it could be cancer of the penis.

ACTION

MAKE AN APPOINTMENT TO SEE YOUR DOCTOR
or go to a clinic for sexually transmitted infections. Any of these skin symptoms may be the result of a sexually transmitted infection, such as genital herpes.

Have you noticed either of the following on your penis?

Flat, painless sore ▶

Small, fleshy lumps ▶

Neither ▶

ACTION

MAKE AN APPOINTMENT TO SEE YOUR DOCTOR
or go to a clinic for sexually transmitted infections. You may have genital warts.

ACTION

MAKE AN APPOINTMENT TO SEE YOUR DOCTOR
if you cannot identify a possible cause for your problem from this chart.

Breast problems

It is important to familiarize yourself with the normal look and feel of your breasts so that you are able to detect any changes in them (see Breasts: self-examination, p.69). Most breast problems are not serious, but consult your doctor if you notice any changes. Minor conditions clearly related to breast-feeding usually respond well to simple treatments.

START

Are you breast-feeding a baby?

Breast-feeding

Not breast-feeding

Where is the problem?

In the breast

On the nipple

What is the nature of your breast problem?

Single lump in the breast

A nipple has changed in appearance

Discharge from the nipple

Breasts feel tender

Breasts feel lumpy and hard

None of the above

What is the nature of your symptoms?

Small, hard lump in breast

Swollen, hard, and tender breasts

Redness of part or all of one breast

None of the above

How is your nipple affected?

Tender only when feeding

Tender and painful all the time

ACTION

MAKE AN APPOINTMENT TO SEE YOUR DOCTOR These symptoms may be caused by minor problems that are easily treatable or that need no treatment. However, such changes must be investigated promptly to rule out the chance of breast cancer.

ACTION

MAKE AN APPOINTMENT TO SEE YOUR DOCTOR Discharge from the nipple may be caused by a local infection or a hormonal problem. However, the possibility of breast cancer needs to be ruled out.

ACTION

MAKE AN APPOINTMENT TO SEE YOUR DOCTOR if you cannot identify a possible cause for your breast problem from this chart.

ACTION

MAKE AN APPOINTMENT TO SEE YOUR DOCTOR if you cannot identify a possible cause for your breast problem from this chart.

ACTION

MAKE AN APPOINTMENT TO SEE YOUR DOCTOR if the lump has not disappeared within a week or if the breast becomes painful or red. The lump may be caused by a blocked milk duct.

ACTION

SEE YOUR DOCTOR WITHIN 24 HOURS You may have mastitis (a breast infection causing inflammation) or even a breast abscess, particularly if you are also feeling unwell.
● Continue to breast-feed from both of your breasts.

ACTION

TRY SELF-HELP MEASURES Overfull breasts are common, especially when you first start breast-feeding and your milk supply has not yet adjusted to your baby's needs.
● Contine to breast-feed your baby at regular intervals.
● Take a painkiller such as paracetamol.
● Place a heated pad or covered hot-water bottle on the affected breast(s).
CONSULT YOUR DOCTOR or breast-feeding adviser if you are concerned.

ACTION

TRY SELF-HELP MEASURES This problem may be a result of your baby not latching on to your nipple properly.
● Make sure that your baby takes the nipple and the surrounding area into his or her mouth properly.
CONSULT YOUR DOCTOR or breast-feeding adviser if you are still having problems when you use the correct feeding technique.

ACTION

TRY SELF-HELP MEASURES Your symptoms may be due to cracked nipples, usually caused by your baby not latching on to your nipple properly.
● Keep your nipples dry between feeds and use moisturizing cream.
CONSULT YOUR DOCTOR or breast-feeding adviser if the problem persists or makes breast-feeding difficult.

Does either of the following apply?

Your next period is due within 10 days

You might be pregnant

Neither

ACTION

MAKE AN APPOINTMENT TO SEE YOUR DOCTOR if you are concerned. The problem may simply be the result of hormonal changes associated with the menstrual cycle that can lead to premenstrual breast tenderness.

ACTION

MAKE AN APPOINTMENT TO SEE YOUR DOCTOR if you cannot identify a possible cause for your breast problem from this chart.

ACTION

MAKE AN APPOINTMENT TO SEE YOUR DOCTOR Breast tenderness is common in pregnancy. If you are not sure whether you are pregnant, do a home pregnancy test.

Painful periods

Many women experience mild cramping pain in the lower abdomen during their periods. This pain is considered normal unless it interferes with everyday activities; it can usually be relieved with painkillers. If you regularly have severe pain or if your periods become more painful than usual, you should consult your doctor to rule out any infections or disorders.

START

Are your periods more painful than usual?

No worse than usual

Worse than usual

ACTION

TRY SELF-HELP MEASURES
Some pain experienced during your period is quite normal.
● Take a painkiller such as ibuprofen.
MAKE AN APPOINTMENT TO SEE YOUR DOCTOR
if pain interferes with normal activities.

ACTION

MAKE AN APPOINTMENT TO SEE YOUR DOCTOR
An increase in period pain is a side effect of some IUDs.

Do you have an intrauterine contraceptive device (IUD)?

IUD

No IUD

Have your periods become heavier or longer as well as more painful?

Heavier

Longer

Neither

Have you had an unusual vaginal discharge between periods?

No discharge

Discharge

Have you had any of the following?

Lower abdominal pain between periods

Low back pain between periods

Fever

None of the above

ACTION

SEE YOUR DOCTOR WITHIN 24 HOURS
You could have pelvic inflammatory disease, in which there is an infection of the reproductive organs.

ACTION

MAKE AN APPOINTMENT TO SEE YOUR DOCTOR
if you cannot identify a possible cause for your painful periods from this chart.

ACTION

MAKE AN APPOINTMENT TO SEE YOUR DOCTOR
You may have fibroids (noncancerous tumours in the uterus) or endometriosis. This is a condition in which the tissue that usually lines the uterus becomes attached to other organs in the abdomen and bleeds during menstruation.

Heavy periods

If you bleed between periods, see p.158 ➤
Some women lose more blood than others during their periods. If normal sanitary protection is not sufficient, bleeding lasts longer than 5 days, or if you notice that you are passing blood clots, the bleeding is probably excessive. If you are concerned about heavy periods, consult your doctor.

START

Are your periods heavier or longer than usual?

About the same

Heavier or longer

Do you have an intrauterine contraceptive device (IUD)?

IUD

No IUD

Have you had a single heavy period that was later than usual?

Yes

No

ACTION
MAKE AN APPOINTMENT TO SEE YOUR DOCTOR
Some IUDs can cause periods to be heavier than normal.

ACTION
MAKE AN APPOINTMENT TO SEE YOUR DOCTOR
Heavy, painful periods may be an indication that you have fibroids (noncancerous tumours in the uterus) or endometriosis, in which the tissue that usually lines the uterus becomes attached to other organs in the abdomen and bleeds during menstruation.

Are your periods more painful than usual?

More painful

The same or less painful

ACTION
MAKE AN APPOINTMENT TO SEE YOUR DOCTOR
Some women regularly have heavy periods, sometimes accompanied by a dragging pain in the lower abdomen. The loss of significant quantities of iron through heavy bleeding could make you susceptible to iron-deficiency anaemia.

ACTION
MAKE AN APPOINTMENT TO SEE YOUR DOCTOR
if you are concerned about the cause of your late period. Late periods may be heavier than usual. However, if you are sexually active there is a possibility that you have had an early miscarriage.

ACTION
MAKE AN APPOINTMENT TO SEE YOUR DOCTOR
if you cannot identify a possible cause for your heavy periods from this chart.

Abnormal vaginal bleeding

Vaginal bleeding is considered abnormal if it occurs outside the normal menstrual cycle, during pregnancy, or after the menopause. Although there is often a simple explanation, you should always see your doctor if you have any abnormal vaginal bleeding. If you are pregnant and you are bleeding, consult your doctor or midwife at once.

Bleeding in pregnancy
If you have any vaginal bleeding during pregnancy, you should contact your doctor or midwife urgently. If the bleeding is heavy, call an ambulance. Although most causes of bleeding are not serious, it is important to rule out miscarriage or a problem such as a low-lying placenta or partial separation of the placenta from the wall of the uterus.

START

Are you pregnant?

More than 14 weeks pregnant

Less than 14 weeks pregnant

Not pregnant

ACTION
CALL YOUR DOCTOR OR MIDWIFE NOW
Bleeding at this stage of pregnancy could be due to a problem with the placenta (see box above right).
● Rest in bed until you receive medical advice.

Is the bleeding similar to that of a normal period?

Like a period

Different

Do you have unaccustomed pain in the lower back or abdomen?

Lower back pain

Abdominal pain

Neither

ACTION
CALL YOUR DOCTOR OR MIDWIFE NOW
You may be having a miscarriage or you may have an ectopic pregnancy.
● Rest in bed until you receive medical advice.

ACTION
CALL YOUR DOCTOR OR MIDWIFE NOW
Bleeding at this stage of pregnancy could be the first sign of a threatened miscarriage.
● Rest in bed until you receive medical advice.

How long has it been since your last period?

Less than 6 months

More than 6 months

Does either of the following apply?

You have only recently started having periods

You are over 40

Neither

ACTION

MAKE AN APPOINTMENT TO SEE YOUR DOCTOR if you are concerned. Irregular periods are fairly common in the first year or so of menstruation.

ACTION

MAKE AN APPOINTMENT TO SEE YOUR DOCTOR if you are concerned or if your pattern does not return to normal within three menstrual cycles. Having an occasional irregular period is unlikely to indicate a serious problem if the period was normal in all other respects.

ACTION

MAKE AN APPOINTMENT TO SEE YOUR DOCTOR if you are concerned. Your periods may become irregular as you approach the menopause.

Hormonal contraceptives

In the first few menstrual cycles after either starting hormonal contraception or changing to a different type of contraceptive pill, spotting is fairly common. If abnormal bleeding persists or develops when there have previously been no problems, you should consult your doctor. He or she may examine you and change the dosage or type of hormonal contraceptive that has been prescribed.

Have you had sex in the past 3 months?

Had sex

Not had sex

Have you noticed bleeding within a few hours of having sex?

Bleeding after having sex

Bleeding unrelated to having sex

ACTION

MAKE AN APPOINTMENT TO SEE YOUR DOCTOR You may have an abnormality of the cervix, such as cervical erosion (in which fragile tissue, which has a tendency to bleed, forms on the surface of the cervix), the development of precancerous cells, or cancer of the cervix.

ACTION

MAKE AN APPOINTMENT TO SEE YOUR DOCTOR Bleeding after the menopause may be due to a minor problem affecting the vagina or cervix, such as cervical erosion (in which the cervix becomes covered with delicate tissue, which has a tendency to bleed). However, the possibility of cancer of the uterus needs to be ruled out.

ACTION

MAKE AN APPOINTMENT TO SEE YOUR DOCTOR if you cannot identify a possible cause for your abnormal bleeding from this chart.

ACTION

CALL YOUR DOCTOR NOW Bleeding, especially if accompanied by pain in the lower abdomen, may be the first sign of an ectopic pregnancy or of an impending miscarriage, even if you were not aware of being pregnant.

Vaginal discharge

◄ If the discharge contains blood, see p.158

A thin, clear or whitish discharge from the vagina is normal. This discharge will vary in consistency and quantity with the stage of the menstrual cycle, during sexual arousal, and during pregnancy. An abnormal discharge is usually caused by infection and should be investigated by your doctor.

ACTION ◄

CONSULT YOUR DOCTOR if you are concerned or if you develop genital irritation. These forms of contraception sometimes cause an increase in normal vaginal secretions.

START ►

What are the characteristics of your discharge?

Thick and white ►

Normal appearance but heavier than usual ►

Greenish yellow ►

None of the above

► **ACTION**

TRY SELF-HELP MEASURES You may have thrush, particularly if you also have genital irritation.

● If you have had these symptoms before, try an over-the-counter product recommended by a pharmacist.

CONSULT YOUR DOCTOR if this is the first time you have had these symptoms.

Do any of the following apply?

You are taking oral contraceptives ►

You have an IUD ►

You are pregnant ◄

None of the above ►

◄ **ACTION**

MAKE AN APPOINTMENT TO SEE YOUR DOCTOR if you cannot identify a possible cause for your discharge from this chart.

Do you have either of the following?

Fever ►

Lower abdominal pain ►

Neither ◄

► **ACTION**

MAKE AN APPOINTMENT TO SEE YOUR DOCTOR if you are concerned or if you develop genital irritation. Increased vaginal secretion is normal in pregnancy.

► **ACTION**

MAKE AN APPOINTMENT TO SEE YOUR DOCTOR or go to a clinic that specializes in sexually transmitted infections. You may have a vaginal infection such as trichomoniasis.

ACTION ◄

SEE YOUR DOCTOR WITHIN 24 HOURS You could have pelvic inflammatory disease (an infection of the reproductive organs).

ACTION ◄

MAKE AN APPOINTMENT TO SEE YOUR DOCTOR Cervical erosion, in which fragile tissue forms on the surface of the cervix, may be the cause of your discharge.

Genital irritation (women)

Itching and/or soreness in the genital area are symptoms of genital irritation, which is often caused by chemicals in toiletries or detergents. Avoid these products and the irritation should clear up. Genital irritation may also be due to infection, but often it has no obvious cause. If the irritation is persistent, consult your doctor.

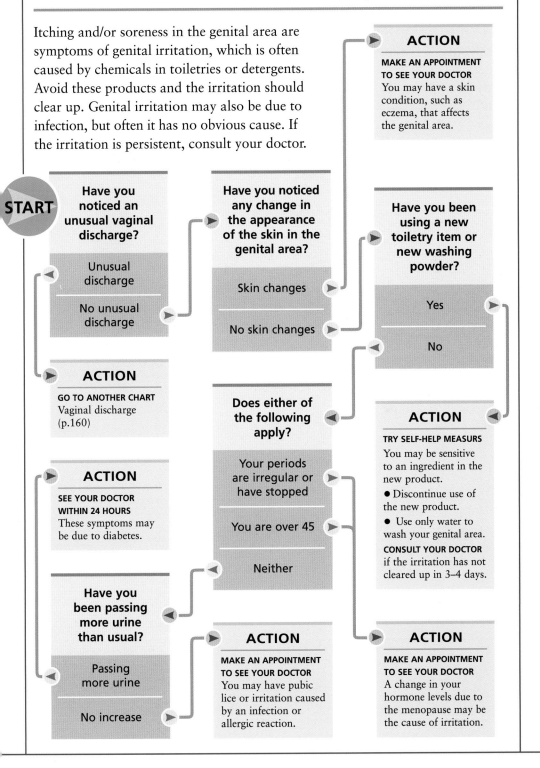

ACTION

MAKE AN APPOINTMENT TO SEE YOUR DOCTOR
You may have a skin condition, such as eczema, that affects the genital area.

START

Have you noticed an unusual vaginal discharge?

Unusual discharge

No unusual discharge

Have you noticed any change in the appearance of the skin in the genital area?

Skin changes

No skin changes

Have you been using a new toiletry item or new washing powder?

Yes

No

ACTION

GO TO ANOTHER CHART
Vaginal discharge (p.160)

Does either of the following apply?

Your periods are irregular or have stopped

You are over 45

Neither

ACTION

TRY SELF-HELP MEASURS
You may be sensitive to an ingredient in the new product.
● Discontinue use of the new product.
● Use only water to wash your genital area.
CONSULT YOUR DOCTOR
if the irritation has not cleared up in 3–4 days.

ACTION

SEE YOUR DOCTOR
WITHIN 24 HOURS
These symptoms may be due to diabetes.

Have you been passing more urine than usual?

Passing more urine

No increase

ACTION

MAKE AN APPOINTMENT TO SEE YOUR DOCTOR
You may have pubic lice or irritation caused by an infection or allergic reaction.

ACTION

MAKE AN APPOINTMENT TO SEE YOUR DOCTOR
A change in your hormone levels due to the menopause may be the cause of irritation.

Home medicine chest

It is a good idea to keep a small supply of medicines at home for everyday aches and pains and first-aid emergencies. Many people now take complementary remedies as well as traditional medicines, and recommendations for both are given here. All medicines should be kept in their original containers with the manufacturer's instructions and stored in a locked cabinet out of children's reach.

CONVENTIONAL MEDICINES

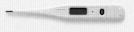

DIGITAL THERMOMETER
Use this type of thermometer for taking a temperature by mouth or armpit

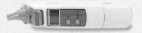

AURAL THERMOMETER
These are used in the ear and are ideal for young children

ORAL SYRINGE
A syringe or dropper is convenient for giving liquid medicines to young children

PAIN RELIEF FOR ADULTS
Paracetamol, aspirin, and ibuprofen give relief from pain and inflammation

ANTACID MEDICATION
Liquid or tablet antacids.can help to relieve the symptoms of indigestion and heartburn

PAIN RELIEF FOR CHILDREN
Liquid paracetamol or liquid ibuprofen give relief from pain, fever, and inflammation

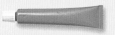

1% HYDROCORTISONE CREAM
Use this cream to soothe itchy or inflamed skin

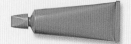

SUNSCREEN
Creams and oils protect skin from sun damage

COLD REMEDIES
Decongestants and lozenges can relieve cold symptoms

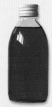

COUGH REMEDIES
Use cough mixtures or lozenges to soothe dry or chesty coughs

ALLERGY MEDICATION
Antihistamines help to control hayfever, allergic conjunctivitis, and bites

ORAL REHYDRATION SACHETS
Mix these sachets with water to prevent dehydration

TRAVEL SICKNESS PILLS
Taking these pills prior to a journey can help to prevent travel sickness

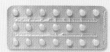

LAXATIVE
Pills or concentrated fruit cubes help to relieve constipation

COMPLEMENTARY REMEDIES

GARLIC

Garlic is a herbal remedy that wards off infection and maintains a healthy heart and circulation

ECHINACEA

Use this herb to protect against infection and to relieve the symptoms of colds, coughs, and 'flu

CHAMOMILLA

This homeopathic remedy soothes teething pains and treats stress, nausea, and vomiting

LAVENDER OIL

This soothing aromatherapy oil eases headaches and aids relaxation

ALLIUM

This is a standard homeopathic remedy for hayfever

ARNICA CREAM

This homeopathic remedy aids the healing of bruises and sprains

VALERIAN

This calming herbal remedy aids relaxation and induces sleep

GRAPHITES

This homeopathic remedy is used to relieve eczema and dermatitis

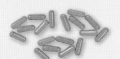

NUX VOMICA

This homeopathic remedy treats indigestion and upset stomachs

USING CONVENTIONAL MEDICINES

- Never give your own prescribed medicines to another person, even if you think that your symptoms are similar.
- Do not use any medicine that is past its sell-by date or that shows signs of deterioration. Dispose of out-of-date medicine by flushing it down the toilet or returning it to the pharmacist.
- Complete the whole course of any prescribed medication, even if your symptoms have gone.

- Never stop taking any prescription medicines unless advised to do so by your doctor.
- Never give a child more than the stated children's dose of a medicine, and never give a child even a small amount of a drug that is intended only for adults, unless advised to do so by a doctor.
- Tell your doctor if you have taken or are taking any homeopathic or herbal remedies.

USING COMPLEMENTARY REMEDIES

- Take homeopathic pillules no less than 30 minutes before or after food, and avoid drinking coffee and eating strongly flavoured foods during a course of medication.
- Ensure that only the person taking the homeopathic remedy touches it, otherwise it may lose its potency.
- Keep the remedies away from any other medications and strong smells.

- Take herbal remedies for short periods only, because the effects of long-term use are not yet known.
- Avoid complementary medicines if you are pregnant or breast-feeding.
- Some remedies may interact with conventional medicines, so consult your doctor before taking a remedy.
- If you have any doubts, consult a homeopath or herbalist for advice.

Caring for a sick person

When looking after any sick person at home, whether a child or an adult, your main concerns will be to ensure that they are comfortable, that they drink plenty of fluids, that they are given the correct medication at the right time, and that any new or worsening symptoms are dealt with correctly. A sick child or baby can be more demanding, but loving, patient care is one of the best aids to recovery.

BRINGING DOWN A FEVER

1 Check temperature

- A fever is a body temperature that is above 38°C (100°F). See pp.68 and 70 for advice on the different ways of measuring a temperature.
- If you or your child develops a fever, look at the charts on pp.74 and 76 to check whether medical help is required or whether the cause can be treated at home.

2 Relieve fever

- Drink plenty of cool fluids.
- Reduce temperature and relieve discomfort with an over-the-counter painkiller such as paracetamol.
- Give babies over 3 months of age and children under 12 years liquid paracetamol (not aspirin).
- Cool young children by removing most of their clothing, wiping them with a facecloth moistened with tepid water, and fanning them, but do not let them get too cold.
- Children under 5 years old are susceptible to febrile seizures (p.43) if they have a high fever and should be watched very closely.

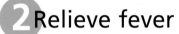

Give cool fluids

Wipe skin with tepid facecloth

Remove clothing and bedclothes

Use fan to keep room cool

SOOTHING A SORE THROAT

- Rest your voice by speaking as little as possible.
- Drink plenty of fluids, especially hot or very cold drinks.
- Eat ice cream and ice lollies; they help ease a tickly throat.
- Take painkillers, such as paracetamol or ibuprofen, in the correct dosages.

- Suck throat lozenges containing a local anaesthetic (these are suitable only for adults).
- Gargle warm salt water (half a teaspoon of salt in a glass of water).
- Install a humidifier or place bowls of water near radiators to keep the air moist.

RELIEVING ITCHINESS

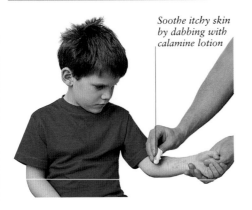

Soothe itchy skin by dabbing with calamine lotion

- For itchiness caused by dry skin, moisturize the skin by applying emollients, such as aqueous cream and petroleum jelly, after washing and bathing.
- To soothe severe itching caused by chicken pox, apply calamine lotion to the spots.
- For severe itching, apply topical corticosteroids sparingly to the area. Always follow the manufacturer's instructions with corticosteroids.

PREVENTING DEHYDRATION

- If you have a fever or are suffering from vomiting and diarrhoea, drink plenty of fluids every 1–2 hours, such as dilute orange juice, weak sweet tea, or an over-the-counter rehydration solution, which contains essential minerals and glucose.
- Do not give milk to adults, children, or bottle-fed babies if they are suffering from diarrhoea or vomiting.
- If a breast-fed baby is affected, continue to breast-feed and offer the baby extra fluids.

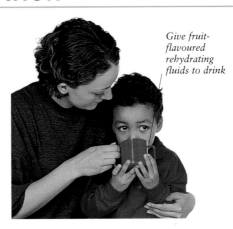

Give fruit-flavoured rehydrating fluids to drink

RELIEVING A BLOCKED NOSE

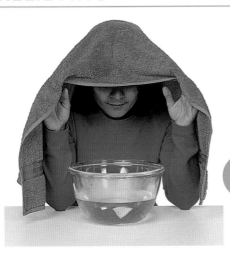

- Fill a bowl or basin with hot water and lean over it with a towel pulled over your head. Breathe deeply.
- Alternative methods are to rub a vapour ointment on to the chest or to use decongestant capsules filled with menthol and other strong-smelling oils to fill the air.

! Important

- Older children should be given steam inhalation only if supervised by an adult.
- Do not give steam inhalation treatment to young children.

ADMINISTERING EYE OINTMENT

To a child

- Wash your hands thoroughly before using the drops.
- Draw the child's lower eyelid away from the affected eye.
- Squeeze a thin line of ointment along the inside of the lower eyelid.
- Ask the child to close the eye briefly.
- Explain that the child's vision may be temporarily blurred.

To yourself

- Wash your hands thoroughly before using the drops.
- Draw your lower eyelid away from the affected eye.
- Squeeze a thin line of ointment along the inside of the lower eyelid.
- Close your eye briefly.
- You may find that your vision is temporarily blurred.

ADMINISTERING EYE DROPS

To a child

- Wash your hands thoroughly before using the drops.
- Sit down and lay the child across your lap, holding his or her head steady. Ask another person to help you if necessary.
- Draw the lower lid away from the affected eye and drop the eyedrops on to the inside of the lower lid, taking care not to touch the eye or the skin around it with the dropper.
- Ask the child to try not to blink straight away.

To yourself

- Wash your hands thoroughly before using the drops.
- Tilt your head backwards and draw the lower lid away from the affected eye.
- Drop the eyedrops on to the inside of your lower lid, being careful not to touch the eye itself or the skin around it with the dropper.
- Try not to blink straight away.

ADMINISTERING NOSE DROPS

To a child

- Lay the child on her back with her head tilted back. Hold her arms, or ask someone to do this for you.
- Hold her head still and drop the nose drops into the nostril.
- Encourage her to sniff up the drops, so that they will be less likely to run out when she sits up.

To yourself

- Lie down on a bed with your head tilted backwards.
- Drop the nose drops into the nostril.
- Sniff up the drop, so that they will be less likely to run out when you sit up.
- Lie still for a few minutes to allow the drops to settle.

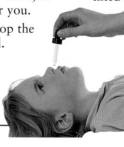

ADMINISTERING EAR DROPS

To a child

- If the drops are being kept in the fridge, allow them to warm to room temperature before using them.
- Lay the child on his side. Hold his head firmly as you squeeze the drops into the ear canal.
- Keep his head still for a minute to allow the eardrops to settle.

To yourself

- If the drops are being kept in the fridge, allow them to warm to room temperature before using them.
- Lie down or tilt your head and squeeze the ear drops into the ear canal.
- Keep your head still for a minute to allow the eardrops to settle.

Hold child's head still

GIVING ASTHMA MEDICATION TO CHILDREN

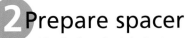

1 Reassure

- Stay calm and reassure the child or baby as he may be frightened by the mask.
- An asthma attack can be frightening not only for the child or baby but also for the adult carer.

2 Prepare spacer

- Check that the inhaler is working by shaking it and depressing it once.
- Place the inhaler in the hole at one end of the spacer.
- Attach the mask (for a baby or young child) or mouthpiece (for an older child) to the other end of the spacer if it is not already in place.

3 Deliver dose

- Sit the child or baby on your lap, place the mouthpiece in the child's mouth or the mask over the baby's face and depress the inhaler.
- Hold the spacer in place until the child or baby has taken five deep breaths, which should be sufficient to inhale all of the drug.

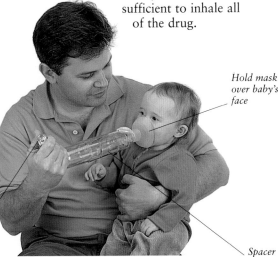

Hold mask over baby's face

Depress inhaler

Spacer

GIVING LIQUID MEDICINES TO CHILDREN

1 Measure dose

- Use a syringe or dropper to avoid spillage and to ensure that you give the correct dose.
- If you are unsure how to use the syringe or dropper, ask your doctor or a pharmacist to show you how to measure and give a dose of medicine to a baby or child.
- Always measure out the dose before you pick up the child or baby, otherwise you may not have enough hands to do the job.

2 Reassure child or baby

- Hold the child or baby securely on your lap to give reassurance and prevent possible struggling.
- Have a drink ready in case the taste is unpleasant to the child or baby.
- If the child or baby is nervous about taking the medicine, explain that the drug will help him feel better and stress that it will all be over very quickly.

3 Place in mouth

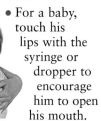

- For a child, place the tip of the syringe or dropper well inside the mouth and angle it towards a cheek.
- For a baby, touch his lips with the syringe or dropper to encourage him to open his mouth.

4 Deliver dose

- Slowly press the plunger or squeeze the dropper, allowing the child or baby time to swallow. Do not aim directly down the child or baby's throat, as this may cause choking.
- If the child or baby spits out the medicine, wait until he has calmed down and then try again.
- Mix the medicine with a little jam, if this helps, but do not add it to a drink because it may stick to the sides of the cup.

DEALING WITH A PANIC ATTACK

1 Calm person

- Stay calm yourself and take the person to a quiet place.

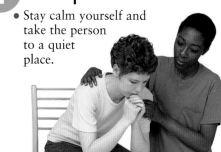

2 Treat hyperventilation

- If the person feels tingling in the fingers, it may be caused by too much carbon dioxide in the blood.
- Encourage her to breathe more slowly. Get her to copy you.
- Try holding a paper bag against her mouth, so that she rebreathes her own expired air, until her symptoms stop.

RELAXATION EXERCISES

1 Get ready

- Performing breathing and muscle relaxing exercises can help rid you of feelings of anxiety.
- Wear comfortable clothing that does not restrict you.
- Choose a warm, quiet room for your relaxation exercises.
- Prepare a firm yet comfortable surface, such as an exercise mat or folded blanket, and have some cushions nearby for extra support.

2 Start with breathing exercises

- Put one hand on your chest and the other on your abdomen.
- Inhale slowly, hold your breath for a moment, then exhale slowly.
- Try to breathe using your abdomen muscles so that the lower hand moves more than the upper hand.
- Once you are breathing from your abdomen, feel your lower hand rise and fall with your abdomen.

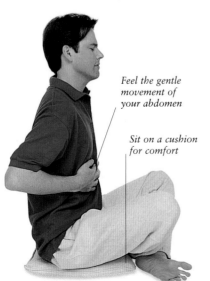

Feel the gentle movement of your abdomen

Sit on a cushion for comfort

3 Relax muscles

- Lie down, put your arms by your side, and let your feet fall open.
- Shut your eyes.
- Take one or two slow, deep breaths. Focus on your breathing.
- Starting with your feet and working up to your head, tense the muscles in each part of your body, hold for a count of three, then release the tension.

Rest your shoulders on the floor

Align your head with your body

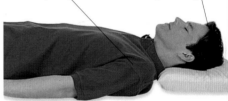

4 Finish by resting

- When you have completed the exercises, lie still for a few moments, keeping your eyes shut, then roll over on to your side.
- Draw your knees up slightly and bend your arms to support your body in a comfortable position.
- After a few minutes, open your eyes and get up slowly.

Use your arms to support your upper body

Rest on a pillow for comfort

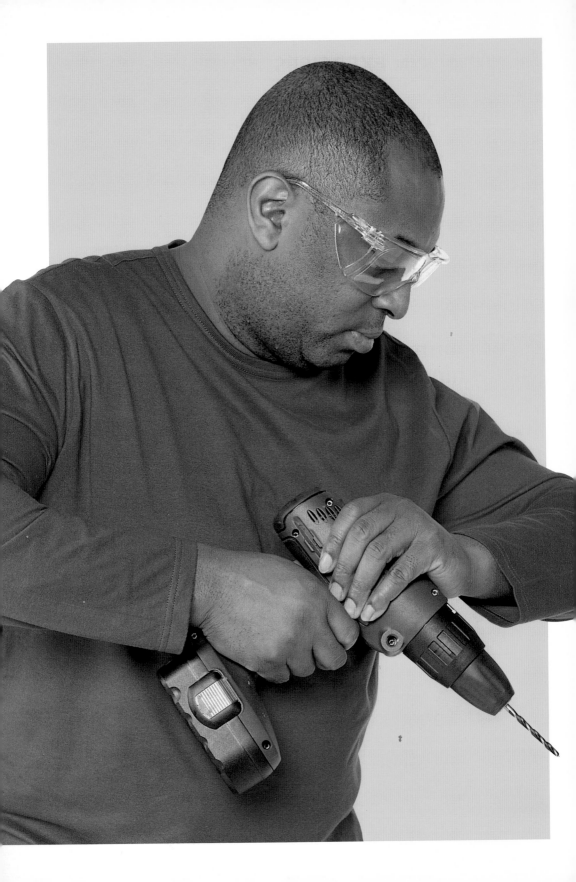

3

DOMESTIC EMERGENCIES

Fires, burst water pipes, blocked sinks, and leaking roofs are just a few of the many domestic incidents that can happen in any home at any time. By knowing how to cope with a wide range of household problems, and having the right equipment for the job, you can minimize any danger to your family and limit damage. Follow the instructions given to fix simple problems yourself, such as bleeding air from a radiator or replacing a pane of glass. For jobs that are less straightforward, learn how to make a temporary fix until you can arrange for a skilled worker to make a permanent repair.

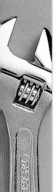

Home safety

Your home should be a place of safety and security, yet every year domestic accidents account for many deaths and countless serious injuries. By being aware of the potential dangers and taking action to make your home as safe as possible, you can do a great deal to reduce the risk of accidents occurring. The following room-by-room guide highlights potential trouble spots and provides practical advice on sensible safety precautions. Most accidents are caused by carelessness, so work safely and wear safety equipment when undertaking do-it-yourself projects.

MAKING YOUR HOME SAFE

1 Be prepared

- Assemble a basic emergency repair kit (see box, right) and keep it in an easily accessible place, such as a wall-mounted cabinet.
- Make sure that all family members know where the equipment is kept.
- Check that any adults know where to find and how to switch off the mains controls for gas (by the gas meter), electricity (by the consumer unit/fusebox), and water (often under the kitchen sink).
- Draw up a family evacuation plan (p.173) and review it regularly.
- Keep a list near the telephone giving numbers for an emergency plumber and electrician, your family doctor, and 24-hour helplines for reporting gas and water leaks.

2 Prepare for fire

- Install smoke and carbon monoxide alarms or detectors (p.173).
- Buy a dry powder fire extinguisher that weighs at least 1 kg (2 lb) and a fire blanket. Keep both near the cooker in the kitchen. Have the extinguisher serviced regularly.
- Buy a flexible metal fire ladder to use when escaping from upstairs.

> **ESSENTIALS**
>
> **EMERGENCY REPAIR EQUIPMENT**
> - First-aid kit (p.60)
> - Torch and spare batteries
> - Lightbulbs
> - Candles and matches
> - Plugs and fuses (p.197)
> - Screwdriver

3 Work safely

- If you are carrying out emergency repairs, take all necessary safety precautions, especially if the work involves electricity.
- Wear the correct safety equipment: safety goggles to protect eyes from flying debris; dust masks to prevent dust from entering the lungs; and ear defenders for use when certain power tools are used in confined spaces.

Wear goggles and a mask to protect against dust

Hold tools firmly for maximum control

MAKING A FAMILY EVACUATION PLAN

1 Plan escape routes

- Decide on the best route for escape – this will usually be your normal way in and out of your home.
- Plan an alternative route to use if the normal way out is blocked.
- If doors or windows need to be unlocked to escape, make sure that everyone knows where to find the keys. Ensure that the doors and windows can be easily opened.

2 Plan meeting point

- Decide on a safe assembly point outside the home where everyone can meet following an evacuation.
- Make sure that the whole family is aware of how to escape and where to meet after evacuation.

3 Practise your plan

- Take a few minutes to walk the escape routes with family members so that everyone knows what to do.
- Practise using these escape routes on a regular basis, especially if you make any changes in your home.
- Wear blindfolds for one practice, to simulate dark and smoky conditions, but be careful with young children and the elderly.

! Important

- Keep escape routes free of furniture and household clutter.
- If you have overnight guests, tell them about your evacuation plan so that they will know what to do in the event of a fire.

INSTALLING SMOKE ALARMS

1 Choose alarms

- Buy battery-operated or electrical alarms that carry the British Standard kitemark and accord with BS5446 Part 1.
- For added safety, choose linked alarms, which set each other off when smoke is detected.

2 Install alarms

- Fix alarms securely into the ceiling at least 30 cm (12 in) away from any wall or light fitting.
- If your home is on one level, fit a smoke alarm in the hall; if it has more than one storey, fit an alarm at the bottom of the stairs and another on each landing.

3 Test regularly

- Check your alarms once a month by pressing the test button. Change the battery in each alarm at least once a year.
- Vacuum the inside of each alarm regularly to keep the sensor chamber free of dust.

INSTALLING CARBON MONOXIDE ALARMS

- Fit one or two carbon monoxide alarms near sleeping areas and in any room with a boiler or a gas fire; these alarms emit a loud noise when they detect the gas.
- Place carbon monoxide detectors next to boilers and gas fires; these detectors change colour if carbon monoxide is present.

MAKING YOUR KITCHEN SAFE

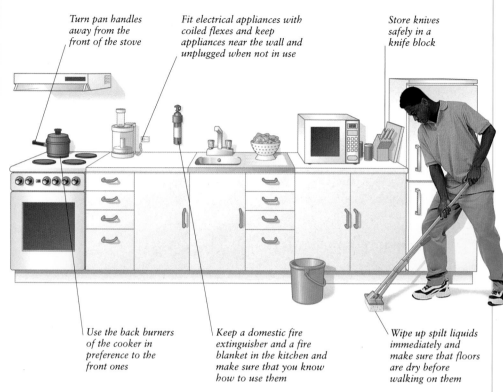

Turn pan handles away from the front of the stove

Fit electrical appliances with coiled flexes and keep appliances near the wall and unplugged when not in use

Store knives safely in a knife block

Use the back burners of the cooker in preference to the front ones

Keep a domestic fire extinguisher and a fire blanket in the kitchen and make sure that you know how to use them

Wipe up spilt liquids immediately and make sure that floors are dry before walking on them

- If you have a boiler in the kitchen, make sure that the flue is kept clear. If you use gas, fit a carbon monoxide alarm in the kitchen or place a detector close to the boiler (p.173).

- Unplug or switch off any electrical appliances at the wall when they are not being used. Kettles, electric carving knives, and kitchen blenders are particularly dangerous items in the wrong hands.

- Use a pair of fold-up steps to reach high shelves instead of standing on a stool, which could cause a fall.

- Never leave a hot chip pan unattended on the stove (p.183).

- Ensure that work surfaces and sinks are well lit so you can work safely.

- If you have young children, fit simple security catches on cupboards and drawers that contain dangerous liquids or sharp knives.

- Store matches, sharp items, and household chemicals well out of the reach of children.

- Try to keep young children out of the kitchen when you are cooking.

- Turn pan handles towards the wall so that children cannot grab them or accidentally knock them.

- Fit guard rails around the stove to keep children away.

- Warn children that cooker tops – especially electric rings, which may show no signs of being hot – can burn even when the power is off.

- Store sharp knives well out of the reach of children, ideally in a wooden knife block.

- Switch off an electric iron and move it out of a child's reach when it is unattended or cooling down.

- Wipe up spills as soon as possible.

MAKING YOUR SITTING ROOM SAFE

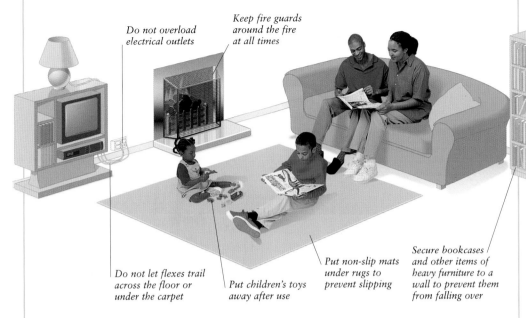

Do not overload electrical outlets

Keep fire guards around the fire at all times

Do not let flexes trail across the floor or under the carpet

Put children's toys away after use

Put non-slip mats under rugs to prevent slipping

Secure bookcases and other items of heavy furniture to a wall to prevent them from falling over

- Avoid running electrical flexes across the floor: these could be tripped over.
- Never run flexes under a carpet where people walk; with wear, bare wires may become exposed.
- Check all electrical wiring regularly: frayed insulation can cause fires.
- Don't overload electric sockets with multi-point adaptors. Use an extension cable with four or six socket outlets instead.
- If you have an open fire, make sure that you use a fire guard, especially when children are present.

- Secure carpets and rugs firmly so that people cannot trip over them. If you have polished wooden floors, place non-slip mats underneath rugs so that they do not move.
- Always check an open fire before going to bed at night and make sure that a fire guard is in place.
- Fit a carbon monoxide detector beside a gas fire (p.173).
- Unplug or switch off electric fires and televisions at the wall socket at night.
- Empty all ashtrays and dispose of the contents safely at night.

MAKING YOUR HALL AND STAIRS SAFE

- Ensure that halls and stairways are well lit – especially if children or elderly people are likely to use them.
- Leave a nightlight on at night.
- If you have young children, fit safety gates at the top and bottom of the stairs and keep them closed.
- Check for worn areas of carpet, which could cause trips or falls.

- Mats and rugs on parquet or polished wood flooring can be dangerous. Place non-slip mats underneath them to prevent them from sliding.
- Install extra grab rails on the stairs to assist elderly people.
- Keep the areas at the top and bottom of the stairs clear at all times.

MAKING YOUR BATHROOM SAFE

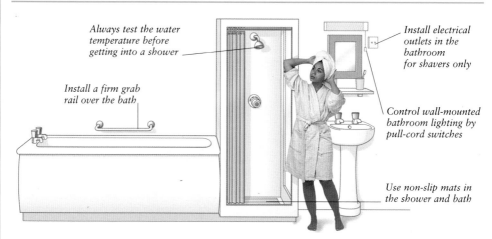

Always test the water temperature before getting into a shower

Install a firm grab rail over the bath

Install electrical outlets in the bathroom for shavers only

Control wall-mounted bathroom lighting by pull-cord switches

Use non-slip mats in the shower and bath

- Fit a grab rail on the wall above the bath rim to provide extra support – especially for elderly people.
- Always run the cold tap first when running a bath for young children.
- Never leave young children on their own in a bath.
- Make sure that any shower unit is fitted with an efficient thermostatic control, so that there is no risk of anyone being scalded.
- Store medicines in a locked cabinet out of the reach of children.
- Never use an electrical appliance, such as an electric fire, hairdryer, or mains radio, in a bathroom.

- Never touch an electrical item with wet hands.
- Make sure that bathroom light fittings and wall-mounted heaters are controlled by pull-cord switches or switches outside the room.
- Check gas water heaters regularly to ensure that flues remain clear. Fit a carbon monoxide detector or alarm (p.173).
- Never mix two types of household chemicals, such as bleach and lavatory cleaner. The combination can produce poisonous fumes.
- Keep all such chemicals out of the reach of children.

MAKING YOUR BEDROOM SAFE

- Service electric blankets regularly and check their wiring for wear and deterioration.
- Never leave electric blankets on overnight unless the instructions make it clear that it is safe to do so. They may overheat and catch fire.
- Keep a small torch and your mobile phone (if you have one) by the bed at night, for use in an emergency.
- Never smoke in bed. You could fall asleep while a cigarette is still alight.

- Never drape a bedside light with a cloth to reduce glare. The heat from the bulb could cause a fire.
- Keep bedroom floors clear of clutter, especially if elderly people or young children are likely to get up to use the bathroom at night.
- If bedroom windows have locks, keep the keys nearby – you may need to use the window as an emergency exit. Leave windows unlocked at night if a room is occupied.

MAKING YOUR CHILD'S BEDROOM SAFE

- Never use pillows or duvets in cots for babies under 1 year old.
- Do not allow very young children to sleep on the upper level of a bunk bed; they may fall out.
- Make sure that there is no gap between mattress and bed rail through which a child could slip.
- When a young child moves out of a cot, fit guard rails to the bed so that she cannot fall out.
- Make sure that there are no lamps within reach of a young child's cot or bed. Bulbs get hot, and pulling on the flex could be dangerous.
- Fit plastic covers over power sockets that are not in use.
- Use plug-in nightlights so that children can find their way if they need to get up in the night.
- Fit removable window restraints so that windows can be slightly opened for ventilation, but fully opened in the event of an emergency.

Put non-slip mats under rugs

Avoid feather pillows and duvets as they can provoke allergies

Keep bedroom floors clear of clutter

MAKING YOUR LOFT SAFE

- Never use free-standing stepladders to get into a loft space: they tend to be unstable and are likely to cause falls. Instead fit a loft ladder with an integral hand rail.
- Fit a light in the loft, preferably controlled from the landing below. Choose a switch that incorporates a light that indicates whether the loft light is on or off.
- Line a loft floor with floorboards, or fix veneered chipboard to the rafters, so that you can store items and move around safely.
- Before storing very heavy items, get a builder or surveyor to check that the rafters are strong enough to support the extra weight.
- Protect ceilings below by distributing the weight of stored items if possible. Put heavier boxes at the sides.

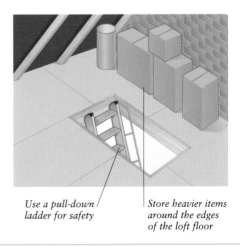

Use a pull-down ladder for safety

Store heavier items around the edges of the loft floor

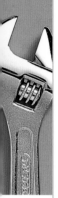

Garden safety

Gardens and outbuildings present many hazards, so safety is an essential part of garden maintenance. Check that garden boundaries are secure, especially if children or animals are likely to be outside, that paths and patios are free of debris, and that outbuildings storing tools and equipment are securely locked. Gardening itself can be a dangerous pastime, so make sure that you also take the necessary precautions when working with tools and machinery.

PREVENTING ACCIDENTS IN THE GARDEN

- Remove or fence off any poisonous plants or trees in your garden.
- Keep children and animals away from any area that has been sprayed with weedkiller.
- Cover outside drains with metal grilles so that children cannot trap their feet inside them. Grilles also help prevent garden rubbish being from being washed into drains and blocking them.
- Fence off ponds, swimming pools, and any other water features in the garden if it is used by children.
- Do not attempt to use a wheelbarrow to move heavy equipment; it will be very unstable. It is far safer to use a low trolley instead.

- Don't risk injuring your back by lifting a heavy load on your own – ask someone to help you.
- Never run a standard domestic mains cable along a fence or bury it below ground when taking power to a shed or workshop. Use special armoured cable underground, or run cable overhead, supported by a special wire. If in doubt, always consult an electrician.
- For garden lighting and water-feature pumps, use a 12-volt system with a transformer and house it in a dry shed or other outbuilding.
- When you are operating electrical power tools, such as lawnmowers or hedge trimmers, always fit a circuit breaker between the piece of equipment and the power source. Always wear the appropriate safety gear, such as safety goggles, protective gloves and if necessary ear defenders.

! Water danger

- Young children can drown in as little as a few centimetres (inches) of water. Even a bucket of water poses a danger.
- If you have a pond, take the precaution of stretching strong plastic netting over the pond and securing it firmly with wooden pegs.
- For complete peace of mind, consider filling in a pond and choosing a safer form of water feature, such as a small fountain.
- Make sure that any water butts have secure lids.

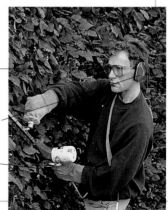

Wear safety goggles to protect eyes

Wear ear defenders if tools are noisy

Choose protective gloves for gardening work

MAKING PATHS AND PATIOS SAFE

- Uneven or broken paving slabs can cause someone to trip and fall. Mend or replace any cracked slabs as soon as possible.

- Icy steps are dangerous. Lay self-adhesive strips of abrasive material on step treads.

- Alternatively, coat the treads with a mix of sharp sand and exterior-grade PVA adhesive.

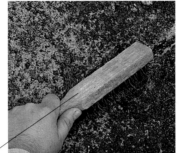

Use a wire brush to remove slippery algae

- During the winter, watch for a build-up of algae slime, which can make surfaces extremely slippery. Clean algae-coated paving with a stiff brush and soapy water, or use a high-pressure washer.

- Prevent algae from building up again by treating the surface with a fungicide.

SECURING BOUNDARIES

- Make sure that garden gates are kept locked and that bolts are well out of the reach of young children.

- If a gate leads on to a road, fit it with a latch that a young child cannot operate. Alternatively, fit a small bolt out of sight on the outside of the gate.

- If you have dogs, or you have young children who use the garden, block off any gaps in hedges or fences through which they could escape.

- Remember that as dogs and children get bigger, a fence may need to be raised and perhaps strengthened.

MAKING GARAGES AND SHEDS SAFE

- Always keep garages, workshops, and sheds securely locked.

- Hang up hoes, rakes, and shovels and store sharp tools, such as saws and knives, and electrical equipment well out of the reach of children.

- Label all dangerous materials and ensure that container lids or caps are firmly closed.

- Store garden chemicals, such as pesticides and fungicides, out of the reach of children, and never tip out-of-date chemicals down sinks or drains. Dispose of them safely.

- Keep chemicals in their original containers and never place them in fizzy drink or squash bottles.

- Never install fluorescent lighting near moving machinery such as lathes. It produces a faint strobe effect that can confuse the senses, making the use of such machinery dangerous.

DO'S AND DON'TS

DO	DON'T
• Use a garage ramp when you are working beneath a car.	• Run a car engine in an enclosed space.
• Wear a dust mask and goggles to protect yourself from dust when sanding.	• Leave a hot soldering iron on a work bench to cool down. Hang it up somewhere out of reach until it is cold.
• Store garden chemicals and tools safely out of the reach of children.	• Leave unattended power tools plugged in or switched on.

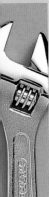

Fires in the home

Statistics reveal that once fire takes hold, you have less than 3 minutes to escape the flames and toxic smoke and get to safety. With such a short time in which to act, it is vital to have organized safe escape routes from your home and to have rehearsed your fire drill with the whole family in advance. Consider installing fire ladders to give you a better chance of escaping from upper floors. If a fire is small, it is worth trying to put it out yourself using water, a fire extinguisher, or a fire blanket. However, if the flames are still burning after 30 seconds, you should leave the building immediately. To give yourself advance warning of a fire, fit smoke alarms on every floor and check them regularly.

ACTION PLAN

START — Are you in the same room as the fire?

Yes ▶

No ▶

Is the fire small?

Yes ▶

No ◀

Have you got a fire blanket or extinguisher that you know how to use?

Yes ▶

No ◀

Have you managed to put out the fire within 30 seconds?

Yes ▶

No ◀

Can you enter the room without risk of danger to assess the fire?

Yes ▶

No ▶

ACTION

EVACUATE THE BUILDING AND CALL THE FIRE BRIGADE (see Escaping from a domestic fire, p.181).

ACTION

OPEN WINDOWS AND DOORS TO CLEAR REMAINING SMOKE.

ESCAPING FROM A DOMESTIC FIRE

1 Alert the family

- A smoke alarm should give you warning of smoke or a fire, or you may see a fire start. Check that everyone in the home is aware of the fire and is leaving quickly.
- Follow the escape route chosen in your evacuation plan (p.173).

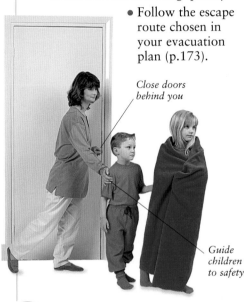

Close doors behind you

Guide children to safety

DO'S AND DON'TS

DO	DON'T
● Feel doors and door handles with the back of your hand before opening them.	● Use lifts.
● Close doors and windows behind you.	● Jump from upstairs windows unless told to do so by fire services or forced by the fire.
● Keep keys by all locked windows.	● Underestimate the speed at which a fire can spread.

2 Evacuate building

- Close internal doors and windows as you go, if possible, to confine the spread of smoke and fire.
- Do not open a door without first touching the door or the handle with the back of your hand to see if it is hot. Heat indicates fire within that room, so choose another route.
- If there is thick smoke, place a handkerchief over your mouth and nose and crawl as low as possible.
- If fire or smoke blocks your escape route, find another way out.
- Once you are out of the building, meet at your agreed assembly point and check that no one is missing.

! If you are trapped upstairs

- Move into a room at the front where rescuers will be able to see you.
- Close the door and wedge a blanket at the base to prevent smoke entering.
- Open a window and shout for help.
- Use a fire ladder if you have one (see box below).

3 Call fire brigade

- Call the fire brigade, state your address clearly, and tell the controller if anyone is still inside the building and if anyone is injured.

USING FIRE LADDERS

- Unfurl and attach the ladder following the manufacturer's instructions. If possible, attach the ladder so that it does not pass over lower windows; otherwise there is risk that you might climb down into flames.
- Help children and the elderly to get on to the ladder and climb down safely. Reassure them and remind them not to look down.
- Use the child harness provided with the fire ladder for a baby or young child.

TACKLING A FIRE

1 Raise the alarm

- Do not attempt to put out a fire yourself unless the fire is small, you discover it early, and you have a fire extinguisher or fire blanket.
- If you have doubts, call the fire brigade and, if necessary, evacuate.

2 Protect yourself

- Make sure that you are able to retreat quickly and safely from the area if the fire gets out of control.
- If the fire is still burning after 30 seconds, evacuate the house at once and call the fire brigade.

USING FIRE BLANKETS AND EXTINGUISHERS

- Take the fire blanket out of its container and give it a shake to open it out.
- Hold the blanket up so that it effectively shields your hands from the fire.
- Drop the blanket on to the flames and leave it there until the fire is out.
- Direct the nozzle of a dry powder fire extinguisher at the base of the flames and sweep it from side to side.

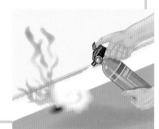

PUTTING OUT CLOTHES ON FIRE

1 Prevent flames rising

- If someone else's clothes are on fire, force the person to the ground so that the flames do not rise up and burn the face and air passage.
- If your own clothes are on fire, lay down immediately to prevent the flames rising up and burning your face and air passage. If you try to run for help, the movement will simply fan the flames.

2 Smother flames

- Wrap the casualty or yourself in a thick wool or cotton blanket, rug, or coat to help smother the flames. Do not use materials that contain synthetic fibres to tackle the fire.
- Roll the casualty or yourself around on the ground until you are sure that the flames are extinguished.

Roll the casualty around to ensure the flames are out

Use a thick woollen rug or blanket to smother the flames

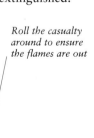

PUTTING OUT AN ELECTRICAL FIRE

1 Switch off power

- Unplug the appliance or, if you cannot safely reach the wall socket, turn off the power at the consumer unit/ fusebox or mains.
- If a computer monitor or television is on fire, there is a risk that the screen could explode: protect yourself by approaching it from the back or the side.

2 Smother flames

- Drape a fire blanket over the appliance to stifle the fire, or douse the flames with a dry powder fire extinguisher (see box opposite).

Place the fire blanket over the burning monitor from behind

PUTTING OUT A CHIMNEY FIRE

1 Douse flames

- Carefully pour water containing detergent on to the fire in the grate. The steam should douse any flames in the flue. Keep pouring until you are sure that the fire is out.
- Ask someone to go outside to check the chimney.

2 Summon help

- If the fire is still burning after you have doused the grate with water, call the fire brigade immediately and evacuate your home.
- Get the chimney is checked and cleared by a chimneysweep before you light another fire in the grate.

PUTTING OUT A CHIP PAN FIRE

1 Approach fire

- Turn off the heat supply.
- Do not attempt to move the pan: the flames may blow back towards you.
- Do not put water on a chip pan fire: the water will disperse the burning fat and so spread the fire.

2 Smother flames

- Cover the flames with a fire blanket (see box opposite). If you do not have a fire blanket, use a towel or tea towel that has been wrung out in water.

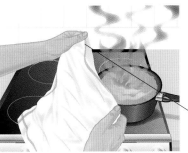

Protect your hands as you approach a burning chip pan

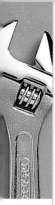

Gas leaks

Natural gas is not poisonous but when combined with air it becomes highly explosive and is capable of destroying a home. Do not attempt to do repairs yourself. This is one of the few areas of domestic maintenance in which any kind of repair or remedial work must be carried out by a nationally registered gas fitter. Because natural gas has no smell, an artificial odour is added to both bottled and mains gas so that leaks can be detected quickly. If you smell escaping gas, you should take immediate action.

ACTION PLAN

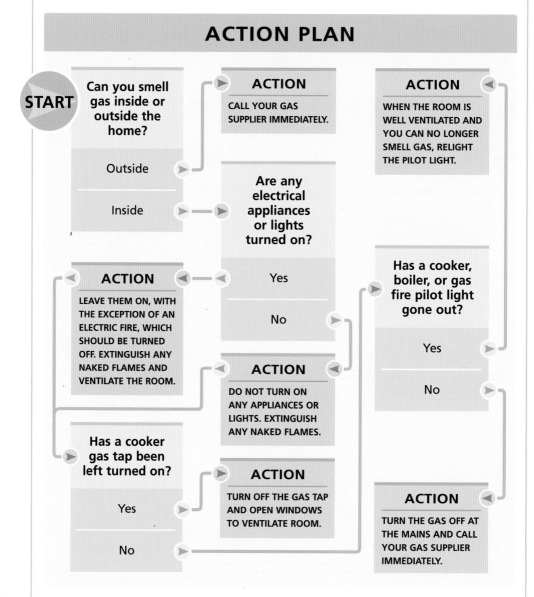

START Can you smell gas inside or outside the home?

ACTION CALL YOUR GAS SUPPLIER IMMEDIATELY.

ACTION WHEN THE ROOM IS WELL VENTILATED AND YOU CAN NO LONGER SMELL GAS, RELIGHT THE PILOT LIGHT.

Outside

Inside

Are any electrical appliances or lights turned on?

Has a cooker, boiler, or gas fire pilot light gone out?

ACTION LEAVE THEM ON, WITH THE EXCEPTION OF AN ELECTRIC FIRE, WHICH SHOULD BE TURNED OFF. EXTINGUISH ANY NAKED FLAMES AND VENTILATE THE ROOM.

Yes

No

Yes

ACTION DO NOT TURN ON ANY APPLIANCES OR LIGHTS. EXTINGUISH ANY NAKED FLAMES.

No

Has a cooker gas tap been left turned on?

ACTION TURN OFF THE GAS TAP AND OPEN WINDOWS TO VENTILATE ROOM.

Yes

ACTION TURN THE GAS OFF AT THE MAINS AND CALL YOUR GAS SUPPLIER IMMEDIATELY.

No

IF YOU SUSPECT A GAS LEAK

1 Avoid danger of ignition

- As soon as you smell gas, or even if you suspect that a gas appliance may be leaking but you cannot smell anything, extinguish any naked flames, such as cigarettes or candles, immediately.
- Switch off any electrical fires.
- Do not touch any other electrical appliances, including light switches. Operating anything electrical could create a spark that could ignite a concentration of gas.

2 Ventilate room

- If you find a gas tap left on, turn it off immediately. Open windows and any external doors.

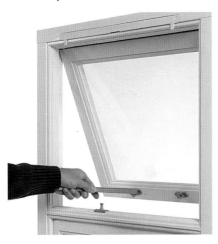

DO'S AND DON'TS

DO	DON'T
• Extinguish any naked flames and cigarettes.	• Turn on any lights or electrical appliances.
• Ventilate the room.	• Use your telephone or mobile phone until you are outside.
• Check gas appliances and pilot lights.	
• Turn off the gas supply at the mains or on the gas cylinder.	• Forget to relight pilot lights once the leak has been mended.

3 Check for leak

- Check all gas appliances and turn off the gas supply at the mains (next to the meter) or on the gas cylinder for bottled gas.
- Send family members outside until the smell of gas has disappeared.

4 Summon help

- If you cannot identify the source of the leak, or can identify it but realize you should not attempt to mend it, evacuate the home.
- Call your regional gas supplier's emergency number from outside your home.
- Keep the family out of the home until the gas supplier advises you that the danger has passed.
- Warn neighbours that you have detected a gas leak.
- Once repairs are complete, do not forget to relight all the pilot lights in the house.

! Carbon monoxide alert

- Alarms to alert you to the presence of carbon monoxide gas can be fitted near boilers or other gas appliances (p.173).
- Carbon monoxide detectors can also be fitted; these work by changing colour when the gas is in the air.

- When the siren sounds or the detector changes colour, ventilate the room by opening external doors and windows.
- Switch off the leaking appliance (or turn off the gas at the mains if you are unsure about the source). Call a gas fitter to repair it.

Plumbing mishaps

Domestic water in the wrong places can cause considerable damage, and the ability to make emergency repairs can prevent a minor problem from becoming a disaster. In a plumbing crisis, it can make all the difference to know the basics, such as where to find your mains stopcock and how to drain the water tank.

ACTION PLAN

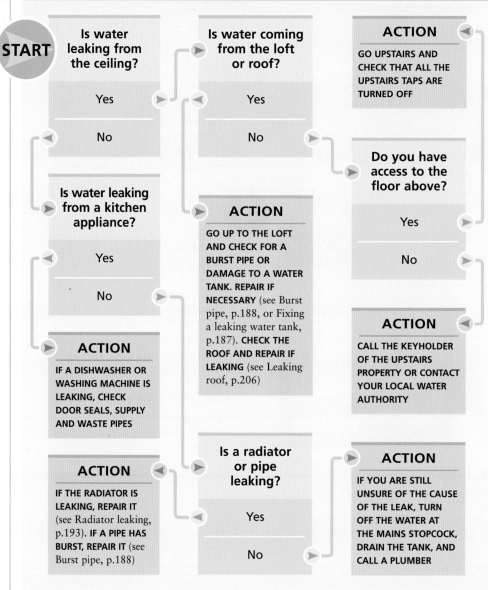

START

Is water leaking from the ceiling?

Yes

No

Is water leaking from a kitchen appliance?

Yes

No

ACTION

IF A DISHWASHER OR WASHING MACHINE IS LEAKING, CHECK DOOR SEALS, SUPPLY AND WASTE PIPES

ACTION

IF THE RADIATOR IS LEAKING, REPAIR IT (see Radiator leaking, p.193). IF A PIPE HAS BURST, REPAIR IT (see Burst pipe, p.188)

Is water coming from the loft or roof?

Yes

No

ACTION

GO UP TO THE LOFT AND CHECK FOR A BURST PIPE OR DAMAGE TO A WATER TANK. REPAIR IF NECESSARY (see Burst pipe, p.188, or Fixing a leaking water tank, p.187). CHECK THE ROOF AND REPAIR IF LEAKING (see Leaking roof, p.206)

Is a radiator or pipe leaking?

Yes

No

ACTION

GO UPSTAIRS AND CHECK THAT ALL THE UPSTAIRS TAPS ARE TURNED OFF

Do you have access to the floor above?

Yes

No

ACTION

CALL THE KEYHOLDER OF THE UPSTAIRS PROPERTY OR CONTACT YOUR LOCAL WATER AUTHORITY

ACTION

IF YOU ARE STILL UNSURE OF THE CAUSE OF THE LEAK, TURN OFF THE WATER AT THE MAINS STOPCOCK, DRAIN THE TANK, AND CALL A PLUMBER

LEAKING CEILING

1 Turn off mains

- Go to the mains stopcock and turn off the water.

2 Drain system

- Turn off the central heating boiler to prevent the pipes overheating.
- Run upstairs cold taps and flush toilets fed by the water tank to reduce the water level in the tank.

3 Release pressure

- Position a bucket to catch water coming from the ceiling.
- If there is a crack, enlarge it with a screwdriver to increase the flow and reduce the weight of water on the ceiling.
- If the ceiling is bulging, put more buckets in place then make a crack.

Enlarge the crack in the ceiling with a screwdriver

> ### ESSENTIALS
>
> **PLUMBING TOOL KIT**
> - Pipe repair tape
> - Plumber's tape
> - Adjustable spanner
> - Sink plunger
> - Mole wrench
> - Plumber's snake
> - Bolt with rubber and metal washers
> - Two-part epoxy resin sealant

4 Find source of leak

- If the water is coming through a ceiling, check the room or the apartment directly above it.
- If the water is coming from the loft area, check for a burst pipe or damage to the water tank and fix any leak (p.188 and below). If the pipes and tank are sound, look for holes in the roof itself and repair if necessary (p.206).

! Dangers of water and electricity

- If water is dripping from a light fitting or on to an electrical appliance, do not touch the fitting or appliance or the controlling switch. Isolate the circuit at the fuse box and call an electrician immediately.

FIXING A LEAKING WATER TANK

- Turn off the water at the mains stopcock.
- Turn on all the cold taps upstairs, and flush toilets fed by the water tank until the tank runs dry.
- If a residue of water remains at the bottom of the water tank, bail it out.
- Plug a small hole by drilling through it and inserting a bolt with rubber and metal washers on either side. For a corner hole, use a two-part epoxy resin sealant.
- Replace the leaking tank with a lightweight polythene tank as soon as possible.

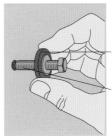

Put rubber and metal washers on both sides of the hole

Insert a bolt into the hole

BURST PIPE

1 Locate frozen pipe

- As water freezes it expands, which can cause old pipes to split open or can push apart a compression joint, where two lengths of copper piping are joined.
- If you have copper pipes, check the compression joints to see if any have been pushed apart.
- If you have lead pipes, look for ice where the pipe wall has cracked.
- Water pipes will freeze only in an uninsulated roof space, outside, or in a house with no central heating.

2 Repair burst pipe

- If the pipe wall is damaged, wrap pipe repair tape around the crack.
- Thaw pipe (see box below) if necessary.
- Call a plumber to make a permanent repair.

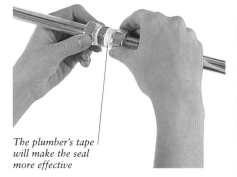

Wrap pipe repair tape around the damaged pipe to seal it

3 Shut off water supply

- If a compression joint is damaged, shut off the water supply to the pipe by closing the gate valve, then repair the joint.
- If the pipe does not have a gate valve, turn off the mains water supply and drain the entire water system by turning on all the taps.

4 Repair joint

- Thaw the joint (see box below).
- Unscrew the joint, wrap plumber's tape around the threaded parts, then refasten the joint.

The plumber's tape will make the seal more effective

THAWING FROZEN PIPES

- If, during winter, you turn on a tap and no water comes out, the pipe may be frozen.
- Find the pipe that feeds the tap, then feel along it until you find the frozen area.
- In addition to feeling very cold, a frozen section of pipe may be bulging under the pressure of the ice.
- Check the pipe carefully for any cracks.

- If there are cracks, then proceed to step 2 above before thawing the pipe. If there are not, thaw it gently.
- Place a hot-water bottle or hot cloths on the pipe or joint, or apply the heat of a hairdryer.
- Do not use a blowtorch to thaw any type of pipework the intense heat is likely cause damage.

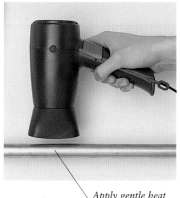

Apply gentle heat to the frozen area

BLOCKED SINK

1 Try sink plunger

- Smear petroleum jelly around the rim of a sink plunger.
- Block the overflow outlet with a piece of cloth, then position the plunger over the plughole. Run 5 cm (2 in) of water into the sink.
- Pump vigorously for a few minutes to clear a minor blockage.
- If this fails, dissolve some washing soda in hot water and pour it down the plughole, or use a proprietary drain clearer.

Block the overflow outlet with a cloth

Pump the plunger over the plughole

CLEAR BOTTLE TRAP

- If the sink is still blocked, place a bucket underneath the bottle trap below the sink and unscrew the base.
- Push a plumber's snake (a flexible length of metal) down the plughole to try to push the blockage out.
- If this is unsuccessful, try working up through the trap bottom and along the waste pipe. Try to pull any debris back towards you rather than pushing it farther away.
- Replace the trap base and fasten securely.

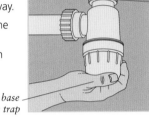

Remove the base of the bottle trap

2 Check U-bend

- For a U-bend with a drain plug (a small capped outlet at the bottom of the U section), put a bucket in place then unscrew the plug using a spanner or wrench.
- Wedge a piece of wood in the U-bend to keep it steady as you work. Clear any debris, then replace the drain plug.
- For a removable U-bend, unscrew the joints and lift out the U section, draining the water into a bucket. Clear debris from the pipe then replace the U section.

3 Check main drain

- If the pipe remains blocked, there could be a problem in the drain.
- Look down each manhole on your property in turn, working from the house out to the road. If you see water pooling in a manhole, this means that the blockage is between that manhole and the main drain in the road.
- Call a drain cleaner to come and clear the drain.

Unscrew both sides of the U-bend to remove blockage

Place a bucket underneath to catch water

LEAKING TAP

1 Turn off water

- A leaking tap is both a nuisance and a waste of valuable water.
- In severe weather conditions, dripping water can freeze in the pipes overnight, which could cause pipes to burst.
- In hard water areas, a tap that keeps dripping may stain sinks and baths with limescale deposits.
- Before starting on any repair work, turn off the water supply.
- Close the gate valve on the pipe, if it has one. If the pipe does not have a gate valve, the only way to cut off the supply is to drain the water tank (Fixing a leaking water tank, p.187).

2 Call plumber

- Most leaking taps are caused by faulty washers.
- You will need to remove the tap cover to replace a washer, which may be tricky if you have modern taps that are complex in design. If feel unsure about tackling the job, ask a plumber to do it.

SILENCING DRIPS

- Until a tap can be repaired, silence the noise by tying a piece of string around its spout. Put the other end of the string in the plughole. The water should now trickle down the string and into the plughole.

AIRLOCK IN PIPE

1 Dislodge air

- If, when you turn on a tap, no water comes out and the pipe makes a banging noise, there is probably an airlock in the pipe.
- You may be able to dislodge the air by using a rubber mallet to tap along the pipe leading from the tap.

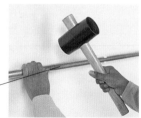

Tap the pipe gently to dislodge the airlock

2 Turn on taps

- If you cannot find the airlock in this way, turn all the taps on full to try to drive out the air.

3 Use garden hose

- If this fails, connect one end of a garden hose to the faulty tap and attach the other end to a mains-fed tap, such as the kitchen sink cold tap.
- Turn on the faulty tap, then the mains-fed one. The pressure of the mains water as it enters the faulty tap should drive the airlock out of the pipe and back up into the water tank.
- When the pipe stops banging, turn off the taps and remove the hose from the mains tap.
- Drain off the water in the hose then disconnect the hose from the faulty tap.
- If airlocks occur repeatedly, the pressure of the mains water supply may need adjusting. Call a plumber to do this job.

BLOCKED TOILET

1 Try to clear toilet

- If the contents of the toilet pan do not flow away when the toilet is flushed, the toilet is blocked.
- Do not keep flushing in the hope that this will remove the blockage: water may build up in the pan and eventually overflow.
- Use a bent wire coat hanger or a plumber's snake to remove a blockage just beyond the bend.

2 Try water force

- If this fails, bail out some water from the pan to reduce the level.
- Try emptying a bucket of water down the toilet. If the blockage is minor, the force of the water rushing down into the pan can be enough to dislodge it.

3 Use plunger

- If the toilet is still blocked, get a toilet plunger or improvise by tying a plastic bag around the head of an old mop.
- Pump the plunger up and down in the pan, but be careful not to use too much force: you risk cracking the toilet pan.
- If the toilet remains blocked, or you prefer not to try any of these remedies, call a plumber.

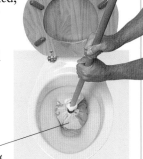

Plunge firmly but carefully so that you do not crack the pan

DRIPPING OVERFLOW PIPE

1 Locate problem

- A dripping overflow pipe from a water tank or toilet cistern means that the correct water level is not being maintained.
- Do not ignore a dripping overflow: the drip could suddenly turn into a serious leak, which could cause a flood, or the water may freeze and result in a burst pipe.
- Look in the water tank or lift the cover of the cistern. Floating on the water is a ball-shaped object attached to the tank or cistern side. This ball float is joined to a float valve, which should close off the supply from the mains when the tank or cistern is full.

2 Check float valve and ball float

- Check the float valve first. If the washer is worn, water will continue to trickle into the tank or cistern even when the ball float has reached its uppermost position.
- Examine the ball float to see if it is leaking. Give it a shake to see whether there is water inside.
- If necessary, buy a new washer or float to replace the faulty one.

3 Call plumber

- If the valve is broken, you will need to call a plumber to mend it.

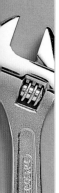

Central-heating problems

Your central-heating system – which comprises the boiler and pump, the radiators, and a header tank – can stop working effectively if a radiator develops a leak or has air trapped in it, or the boiler pump jams. Dealing with these problems is usually straighforward. Use the action plan below to identify the fault, then follow the instructions on the opposite page to remedy it. Alternatively, call a plumber or central-heating engineer.

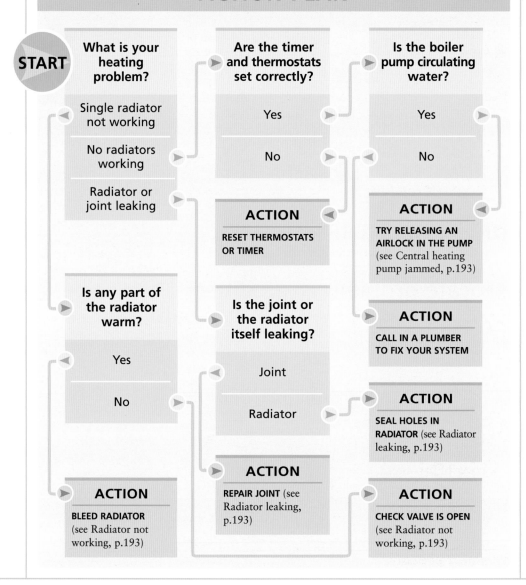

ACTION PLAN

START

What is your heating problem?

Are the timer and thermostats set correctly?

Is the boiler pump circulating water?

Single radiator not working

Yes

Yes

No radiators working

No

No

Radiator or joint leaking

ACTION

RESET THERMOSTATS OR TIMER

ACTION

TRY RELEASING AN AIRLOCK IN THE PUMP (see Central heating pump jammed, p.193)

Is any part of the radiator warm?

Is the joint or the radiator itself leaking?

ACTION

CALL IN A PLUMBER TO FIX YOUR SYSTEM

Yes

Joint

No

Radiator

ACTION

SEAL HOLES IN RADIATOR (see Radiator leaking, p.193)

ACTION

BLEED RADIATOR (see Radiator not working, p.193)

ACTION

REPAIR JOINT (see Radiator leaking, p.193)

ACTION

CHECK VALVE IS OPEN (see Radiator not working, p.193)

RADIATOR NOT WORKING

1 Check valve
- Check that the valve at the bottom of the radiator is fully open.

2 Check thermostats
- Look at the main central heating thermostat and the radiator's own thermostat (if present) to check that both are set correctly.

3 Bleed radiator
- Fit an air bleed key into the air bleed valve at one end of the top of the radiator.
- Hold a cloth underneath the valve and turn the key anti-clockwise until you hear air hissing out.
- Turn the key clockwise as soon as water, which may be hot, starts dripping out.

RADIATOR LEAKING

1 Find leak
- Pinpoint the source of the leak. Water can escape through a loose joint between the pipe and radiator; or through one or more tiny holes in a radiator caused by corrosion.

2 Repair joint
- Tighten the nut with a spanner.
- If water still leaks, turn off the heating and call a plumber.

3 Seal small hole(s)
- Add a liquid radiator sealant to the header tank (a small cold water expansion tank in the loft).
- Run a hosepipe from the central heating draincock (usually under the boiler or on the last radiator in the system) to a drain or sink, then drain the system. The sealant flows through and seals the leak.
- The sealant is only a temporary repair, so replace the radiator soon.

CENTRAL HEATING PUMP JAMMED

1 Find valve
- Turn off the central heating pump (this will be sited near the hot water tank) and find the bleed valve.
- Place a screwdriver in the bleed valve and have a cloth ready to catch the water that will be released when the airlock is released.

2 Release airlock
- Expel any air from the pump in the same way as bleeding a radiator (see above).
- If the pump is still jammed, call a plumber or central heating engineer.

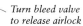

Turn bleed valve to release airlock

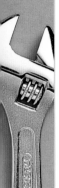

Air-conditioning problems

There are two main types of air conditioning, whole-house systems and single-room units. Both circulate clean air that is cool in the summer and warm in the winter. Problems with whole-house air conditioners are best dealt with by an air-conditioning specialist, but basic maintenance of single-room units, such as checking thermostat settings, cleaning the filter, repositioning the sensor, and cleaning the condenser, is usually straightforward and you can do it yourself.

ACTION PLAN

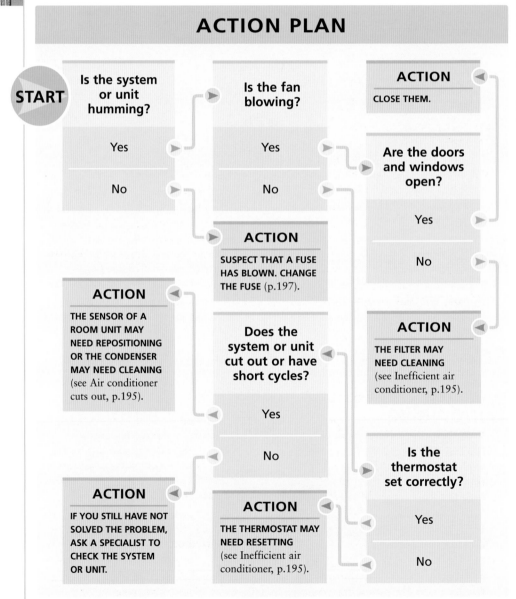

START

Is the system or unit humming?

Yes

No

Is the fan blowing?

Yes

No

ACTION

CLOSE THEM.

Are the doors and windows open?

Yes

No

ACTION

SUSPECT THAT A FUSE HAS BLOWN. CHANGE THE FUSE (p.197).

ACTION

THE SENSOR OF A ROOM UNIT MAY NEED REPOSITIONING OR THE CONDENSER MAY NEED CLEANING (see Air conditioner cuts out, p.195).

Does the system or unit cut out or have short cycles?

Yes

No

ACTION

THE FILTER MAY NEED CLEANING (see Inefficient air conditioner, p.195).

Is the thermostat set correctly?

Yes

No

ACTION

IF YOU STILL HAVE NOT SOLVED THE PROBLEM, ASK A SPECIALIST TO CHECK THE SYSTEM OR UNIT.

ACTION

THE THERMOSTAT MAY NEED RESETTING (see Inefficient air conditioner, p.195).

INEFFICIENT AIR CONDITIONER

1 Reset thermostat

- If the air conditioner is switched on but the fan is not blowing, check the temperature setting on the thermostat. If the thermostat is set too high for the current conditions, the air conditioner will not be stimulated to operate.
- Reset the thermostat to a lower temperature. The fan should start to work straight away.

2 Remove filter

- If the fan is working efficiently but the room or house is still too warm, the filter may need either cleaning or replacing (depending on the type of air conditioner).
- For a whole-house system, ask an air-conditioning specialist to clean or replace the filter, as appropriate.
- For a single-room unit, unplug the unit at the wall. Remove or lift up the front panel, depending on the design, and remove the filter.

3 Clean filter

- Clean the filter with some warm water containing a mild detergent then rinse it in clean water and dry it thoroughly.
- Replace the filter and turn the unit back on.

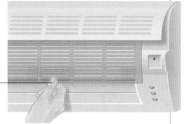

Clip filter back into place after cleaning

4 Fit new filter

- If your unit has a disposable filter, check its condition. If it has turned black, is warped, or has holes in it, then it needs replacing.
- Remove the old filter and fit a new one, following the manufacturer's instructions. Then replace the front panel, and turn the unit back on.

AIR CONDITIONER CUTS OUT

1 Reposition sensor

- For a single-room unit, unplug the unit at the wall. Remove the front panel and filter.
- Check the thermostatic sensor; it should be near, but not touching, the evaporator coils. Move it away from the coils if necessary.
- Replace the filter and front panel and plug the unit in.
- For a whole-house system, get an air-conditioning specialist to reposition the sensor for you.

2 Clean condenser

- For a wall-mounted single-room unit, remove the condenser (the part of the unit outside the room) first. The condenser in a window-mounted single-room unit can be cleaned in situ.
- Use a vacuum cleaner to remove all the dust and lint that has collected on the condenser.
- For a whole-house system, get an air-conditioning specialist to clean the condenser for you.

Electrical problems

We all take electricity for granted – flick a switch and a light comes on, plug the television in and it works – but fuses can blow, electrical equipment can go wrong, and wirings and fittings can become damaged or overheated, posing a potential fire hazard. By equipping yourself with some basic electrical knowledge, you will be able to rectify common problems quickly when they occur.

ACTION PLAN

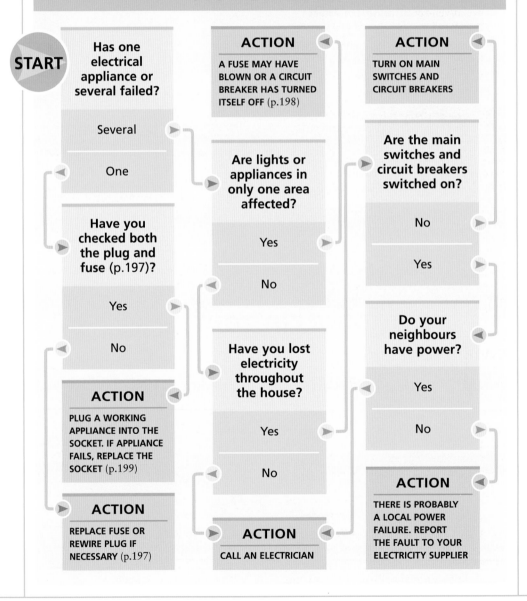

START

Has one electrical appliance or several failed?

Several ▷

One

Have you checked both the plug and fuse (p.197)?

Yes ▷

No ◁

ACTION

PLUG A WORKING APPLIANCE INTO THE SOCKET. IF APPLIANCE FAILS, REPLACE THE SOCKET (p.199)

ACTION ◁

REPLACE FUSE OR REWIRE PLUG IF NECESSARY (p.197)

ACTION ◁

A FUSE MAY HAVE BLOWN OR A CIRCUIT BREAKER HAS TURNED ITSELF OFF (p.198)

Are lights or appliances in only one area affected?

Yes ▷

No ◁

Have you lost electricity throughout the house?

Yes ▷

No ◁

ACTION ◁

CALL AN ELECTRICIAN

ACTION ◁

TURN ON MAIN SWITCHES AND CIRCUIT BREAKERS

Are the main switches and circuit breakers switched on?

No ▷

Yes ▷

Do your neighbours have power? ◁

Yes ▷

No ▷

ACTION ◁

THERE IS PROBABLY A LOCAL POWER FAILURE. REPORT THE FAULT TO YOUR ELECTRICITY SUPPLIER

FAULTY APPLIANCE

1 Check plug

- Loosen the large screw between the pins and remove the plug cover.
- Check the wiring inside the plug for loose connections.
- Check that each wire is securely attached to the correct terminal – brown to Live, blue to Neutral, and green/yellow (if present) to Earth (see Rewiring a plug, below).
- If the plug is a sealed unit, you will have to call an electrician to check why the appliance is not working.

2 Check fuse

- Check that a fuse with the correct amperage is fitted (3A for items such as clocks, fridges, lamps, and televisions, 5A for items such as hi-fi systems, and 13A for items such as kettles, dishwashers, hairdryers, and lawn mowers).
- If the fuse is blown, replace it with one of the correct amperage.
- Tighten the cord grip screws and refit the plug cover.
- If the appliance still does not work, try the plug in another wall socket.

DO'S AND DON'TS

DO

- Turn off appliances at the wall socket when not in use.
- Switch off the wall socket and remove the plug before you attempt to repair an appliance
- Have your wiring checked by a professional at least once every 5 years.

DON'T

- Touch plugs, sockets, or switches if your hands are wet.
- Fit a fuse of the wrong amperage in a plug: you risk electrocution or even fire.
- Attempt electrical work unless you are confident that you know what to do.

REWIRING A PLUG

- Remove the plug cover, loosen the terminal screws, and ease out the flex.
- Position the flex on the plug with the wires placed in their correct positions to gauge whether you need to remove any of the outer insulation on the flex.
- If necessary, use wire strippers to cut away 50 mm (2 in) of the outer insulation, then reposition the flex.

- Cut each wire to length (each one should be long enough to reach its terminal) and use wire strippers to remove 6 mm (¼ in) of insulation from the end of each wire.
- Replace the flex in the plug, fit the cord grip loosely, and push each wire carefully into its terminal.
- Tighten each terminal screw down on to its wire and refit the plug cover.

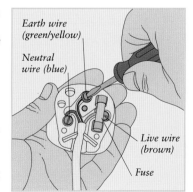

Earth wire (green/yellow)

Neutral wire (blue)

Live wire (brown)

Fuse

ELECTRICAL CIRCUIT FAILURE

1 Find blown fuse

- If power fails in one part of the home, affecting several appliances and lights at once, go to your consumer unit/fuse box.
- If your unit has miniature circuit breakers (MCBs), look for one in the "off" position and simply flick it back on, or push the reset button.
- If the unit has either rewirable or cartridge fuses, switch off the main switch and remove the unit's cover.
- For rewirable fuses, unplug each fuse until you find the one in which the wire has broken or melted.
- With cartridge fuses, you will need to test each fuse by replacing it with one of the same amperage and seeing if the circuit works.

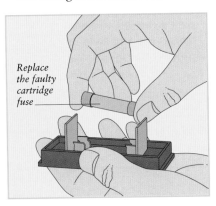

Replace the faulty cartridge fuse

2 Fix rewirable fuse

- Loosen the two terminals holding the burnt wire and remove it.
- Select a new length of the correct type of fuse wire (5A for lighting, 15A for immersion heaters, 30A for wall sockets, and 45A for cookers).
- If the wire does not have to pass through a tube in the fuse carrier, wrap one end of it clockwise round one of the terminals, then tighten the screw. Take the wire across to the other side and attach it to the other terminal in the same way.
- If the wire does pass through a tube in the fuse carrier, insert the new wire before wrapping it around both terminals.

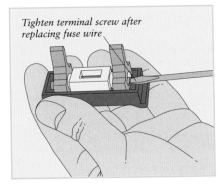

Tighten terminal screw after replacing fuse wire

! Replacing fuse wire

- Do not use fuse wire that is heavier than the gauge intended for the circuit. This could lead to a dangerous fault going unnoticed because the fuse wire will fail to melt; if there is a fault, the fuse wire will not "blow", which could result in a fire.
- Never use any other type of wire or metal strip as a substitute for fuse wire.

3 Identify recurrent fault

- If the MCB switch will not stay in the "on" position, or the fuse blows again when you turn the power back on, try to identify the fault.
- Check to see whether any light bulbs have blown, then switch off all appliances on that circuit and switch them back on one at a time.
- If you cannot find the cause of the problem, call an electrician.

FAULTY WALL SOCKET

1 Look for signs of damage

- Check for any scorch marks on a socket or round the base of plug pins – these show poor connections.
- If you have already checked or fixed the plug (p.197), and the appliance works in another socket, the socket is probably faulty and will need to be replaced.
- If any part of the socket is wet, do not attempt to replace it – ask an electrician to do it for you.

2 Replace socket

- If possible, buy a new socket that is identical to the old one so the wires will be in the same place.
- Switch off the power at the consumer unit/fuse box and take out the relevant fuse (or flip the switch to the "off" position if your unit has MCBs).
- Remove the fixing screws from the socket and pull it out of its box. Make a note of which wires lead to which socket terminals.
  - Loosen the terminals to free the conductor wires, then connect the wires to the correct terminals of the new socket.
  - Put the new socket into the old box and screw it in place.

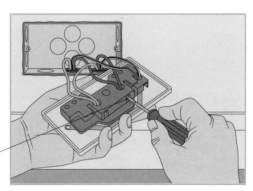

Reconnect the wires to the new socket

WORN ELECTRICAL FLEX

1 Look for signs of damage

- If the sheathing on an electrical flex is damaged or worn, you could be electrocuted if you touch the exposed inner wires.

2 Check inner wires

- Unplug the flex at the wall.
- If the inner wires are damaged, do not use the appliance until an electrician has replaced the cord.

3 Make repair

- If the inner wires are undamaged, wrap insulating tape around the flex as a temporary measure until an electrician can replace the cord.

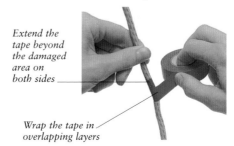

Extend the tape beyond the damaged area on both sides

Wrap the tape in overlapping layers

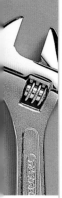

Structural problems

The majority of structural problems can be prevented by giving your home a regular internal and external maintenance check. Look at the condition of your windows, doors, roof, walls, fences, and drains, and deal with minor defects immediately before they become major problems. Even in a well-maintained home, however, there is plenty that can go wrong – windows get broken, doors stick, roof tiles fall off, and holes appear in guttering – but the advice here will help you to make at least a temporary repair before seeking expert advice.

SECURING BROKEN PANE OF GLASS

❶ Make cracks safe

- If the glass is cracked, cover the crack(s) with clear, self-adhesive waterproof repair tape on both sides of the glass to hold it in place temporarily.
- Either replace the pane yourself (see opposite) or get a glazier to do the job for you.

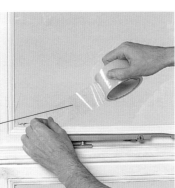

Tape over the cracks carefully to avoid breaking the glass

❷ Cover shattered pane

- If the glass is shattered, cover the outside of the hole with a sheet of polythene and secure it to the frame with battens and pins or strong tape.
- For greater security, screw a sheet of 12-mm (½-in) thick plywood over the inside of the broken door or window pane.
- If you feel that you can do the job, replace the glass yourself (p.201), otherwise ask a glazier to do it for you.

CHOOSING AND MEASURING FOR REPLACEMENT GLASS

- Safety glass is reinforced in manufacture and must be used when glazing a very large area, such as a patio door or picture window, where it could be mistaken for an opening, or where glass will be fitted within 80 cm (31 in) of the floor.
- There are three types of safety glass: toughened glass, laminated glass, and wired glass. If you need to use safety glass, discuss with your glass merchant which type is most suitable for the window or door in question.
- If the glass is patterned, take a piece to match with the new glass.

- Measure the height and width of the opening, going right into the groove cut for the glass in the frame. Cut away any old putty or remove old beading to make sure. Since the cavity may not be square, take two measurements on each dimension and use the mid-point as your figure.
- Measure the two diagonals of the opening. If they are not the same, make a cardboard template to give to your glass supplier.
- Buy a pane of glass that is 3 mm (⅛ in) smaller than the cavity on each dimension; also buy some putty and some glazing sprigs.

REPLACING DAMAGED PANE OF GLASS

1 Remove old glass

- Put on strong protective gloves and safety glasses.
- If the glass is only cracked, run a glass cutter around the edge about 25 mm (1 in) from the frame. Place self-adhesive tape across the cracks, then tap the glass with a hammer. It should come away in one piece.
- If the glass is shattered, sweep up the debris, then lever out any loose pieces still in the frame. Use an old chisel and hammer to remove pieces from around the edges, with the old putty. Work from the top of the frame downwards.
- Use pincers to extract the glazing sprigs (the tiny nails used to hold the glass in place), then brush the frame to remove small fragments.
- Dispose of the broken glass safely.

2 Insert new glass

- Wet your hands and then knead some putty to make it pliable. Working on the outside of the window, press a continuous putty line all around the edge where the glass will rest using your thumb.
- Place the glass, lower edge first, on to the putty and press it firmly into place, leaving a 3-mm (⅛-in) gap all around.

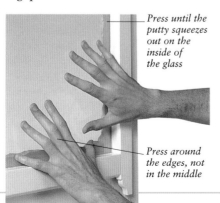

Press until the putty squeezes out on the inside of the glass

Press around the edges, not in the middle

3 Secure new glass

- Fix the glass into position with glazing sprigs spaced about 20 cm (8 in) apart. Tap them gently into the frame with a small hammer, ideally a pin hammer.

Keep the hammer head parallel to the pane of glass

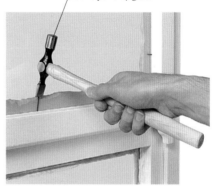

- Remove any surplus putty on the inside edge of the glass with a wet putty knife (a small, pointed, wide-bladed knife).
- Roll some more glazing putty into a thin sausage and press it into the join between glass and frame all around the outside of the window.
- Smooth it by holding the putty knife at a 45° angle to the frame, with the flat of its blade on the putty, and pulling it along. Mitre the corners.
- Leave the putty to dry for at least 2 weeks before painting.
- If the glass is held by beading, apply a strip of self-adhesive plastic foam around the outside edge of the glass before pinning on the beading.
- Repaint the frame, taking a 3-mm (⅛-in) margin of paint on to the glass to ensure that rainwater will not get behind the putty and into the wood frame.

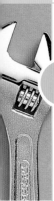

DOORS AND WINDOWS THAT STICK

1 Remove paint layers

- A build-up of paint layers can cause doors and windows to stick.
- Strip off all the paint back to bare wood, then repaint.

2 Plane door

- If a door or window catches as you close it, take it off its hinges, plane a little off the top, bottom, or side, depending on where it catches, then rehang it.

Plane to bare wood on the edge that is sticking

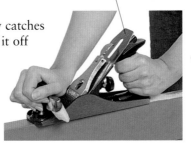

3 Prevent dampness

- A door that is sticking in damp weather but fits perfectly well in dry weather is absorbing moisture, probably through an unpainted top or bottom edge. Ideally, wait for dry weather before painting it.
- If the bottom edge of a door is unpainted, you will have to take the door off its hinges before you paint and rehang it.
- If this does not solve the problem, plane the sticking edge, smooth it with sandpaper, if necessary, then paint and rehang as before.

DAMAGED WINDOW JOINTS

1 Make temporary repair

- Joints that shrink as the wood dries out can cause a window to sag.
- A sash window will need to be removed for repairs (see step 2).
- A prominent casement window can be temporarily repaired in situ until you have time to make a permanent repair (see step 2). If the window is not in a prominent position, most repairs can be done in situ.
- Unscrew the frame a little and then prise the loose joint open slightly. Squeeze some PVA woodworking adhesive into the gap.
- Screw an L-shaped metal bracket across the joint to hold it together.

2 Make permanent repair

- For a permanent, and more sightly, repair, remove the window and unscrew the frame.
- Prise the loose joint open and squeeze some PVA woodworking adhesive into the gap.
  - Hold the joint in an adjustable sash clamp until it has set, then replace the window.

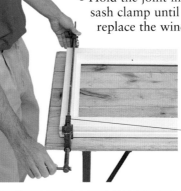

Place the joint in a sash clamp and leave until the adhesive has dried

DAMAGED SASH WINDOWS

1 Ease sticking parts

- If a sash window sticks a little, rub a candle on to the sliding parts and put oil on the pulleys.
- If the window is sticking badly, it is likely that a joint has dried out and needs repairing (p.202).

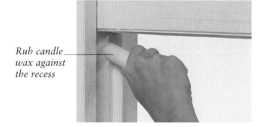

Rub candle wax against the recess

2 Damaged or broken sash cords

- If the sash cords have broken, so that the top window crashes down, you will need to get them replaced.
- In the meantime, you can make the window safe by using lengths of wood to wedge it shut.
- Replacing sash cords is not easy because replacement cords must be fitted with the correct weights in order to balance the weight of the sash windows, including the glass. Get a window repairer to do the job for you.

BADLY FITTING HINGES

1 Replace protruding screws

- Check the hinge screws. If the heads are protruding, a door or window will not close properly against the frame. Try screwing them in more tightly.
- If this is unsuccessful, replace any protruding screws with smaller-diameter, longer screws.

2 Pack out hinge

- If a hinge is recessed too far into the frame, the door or window will not close properly.
- Take the door or window off its hinges and remove the hinge.
- Pack out the recess with a piece of card the same size as the hinge.
- Replace the hinge and rehang the door or window.

3 Tighten screws

- If a hinge is too loose, the door or window will not hang properly. Tighten loose screws or replace them with longer screws.

4 Recess hinge

- If a hinge is insufficiently recessed into the frame, the door or window will not close properly.
- Take the door or window off its hinges and remove the hinge.
- Use a wood chisel to carefully cut a deeper recess for each affected hinge, then replace the hinge.

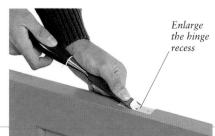

Enlarge the hinge recess

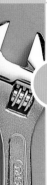

DEALING WITH WOOD ROT

1 Assess damage

- Rotten wood at the foot of doors or around window frames is usually caused by wet rot.
- Wet rot occurs when timber gets damp, often when water has seeped through damaged paintwork. A first sign is often peeling paintwork.

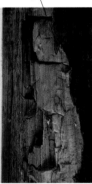

A sign of wet rot is timber that is dark brown and crumbly when dry

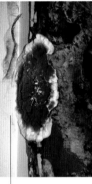

A cotton-wool like material and rust-coloured spores indicate dry rot

- If you can detect a strong, musty, mushroomy smell indoors, or see a white, cotton-wool like material below skirting boards or through floorboards, you may have dry rot.
- Dry rot affects timber in badly ventilated confined spaces, and it spreads rapidly. Call in rot treatment specialists immediately.

2 Treat cause of wet rot

- Before repairing damaged wood, try to find out why the wood has become damp. Check for a leaky pipe or blocked drain.
- Fix the cause of the damp and leave the wood to dry out.

3 Cut away damaged wood

- Chisel out all the decaying material until you reach sound, solid wood.
- Coat the sound wood and surrounding woodwork with a chemical wet rot eradicator.

4 Apply wood hardener

- Brush a coat of wood hardener on to the exposed wood. This varnish-like liquid binds the loose fibres of wood together and seals the surface, making it ready for replacement wood or filler.

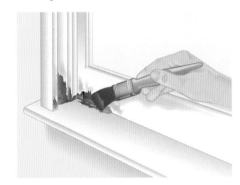

5 Fill hole

- For extensive damage, use new wood, treated with preservative, to fill the main gap.
- For smaller gaps, use a special two-part wood filler, following the manufacturer's instructions. Use wood filler also to fill any gaps around new wood.
- Once the filler is dry, rub it down with glass paper until smooth, then paint, stain, or varnish.

BROKEN OR UNSTABLE FENCING

1 Replace panel

- If a fence panel has been damaged by an impact, blown over by high winds, or is in a state of disrepair, you will need to replace it.
- For a panel supported by timber posts or recessed concrete posts, remove the nails or angle brackets holding the panel in place at each end and remove the panel. Hold a new panel in place and reattach it.
- For a panel supported by grooved concrete posts, slide the old panel out and slide a new one in.

Slot the fence panel into the grooved concrete post

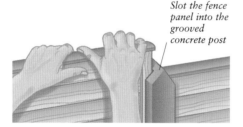

2 Replace post

- If a fence post wobbles, it is rotten at the base and needs replacing.
- Detach the fencing on either side. If the fence is closeboarded, wedge strong timber props under the top edge to hold the fence in place while you work on the post.
- For a post set in concrete, cut it off at ground level, drive a metal repair socket into the centre of the stump, then insert a new post cut to the right length. Reattach the fencing panels on either side.
- For a post not set in concrete, dig it out and replace it with a new one.
- Before inserting the new post, soak it in chemical preserver overnight to protect it against rot.
- Anchor the new post firmly into the ground then reattach the fencing panels on either side.

BROKEN OR UNSTABLE GATE

1 Replace post

- A rotten gate post should be replaced by a new wooden post (see Replace post, above).

2 Make gate stable

- If a gate is generally unstable, check the diagonal brace on the back of the gate. If this is not sound, replace it with a new one.
- Alternatively, if a joint is loose, open the joint slightly and squeeze some waterproof adhesive into it. Use a metal bracket to keep the joint together, fixed with 25-mm (1-in) galvanized or alloy screws.

3 Secure hinges

- If a gate is sagging, the hinges may need to be secured using longer or thicker screws.

Reattach the hinges with stronger screws

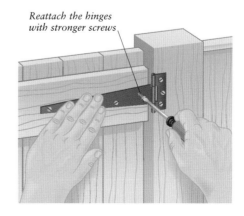

LEAKING ROOF

1 Inspect the roof

- Look at your roof from the ground, using binoculars if necessary, to see if you can spot any slipped or missing tiles or slates.
- Go into the loft with a torch and inspect the roof from the inside.
- If the roof is lined, check the lining for damp stains.
- If the roof is unlined, look for chinks of daylight between tiles.
- Check the roof timbers for damp.
- If the source of the leak is at a junction between the roof and other parts of the building, such as a wall or chimney, inspect the metal strips (flashing) that seal the join from the outside.
- Once you have identified the source of the leak, make a temporary repair from inside (see box) if you can, then call a roofing contractor to make a permanent repair.

2 Remove tiles/slates

- Wedge up the tiles or slates that overlap the damaged one, then rock it loose and slide it out carefully.
- Buy a matching tile or slate from your local builder's merchants.

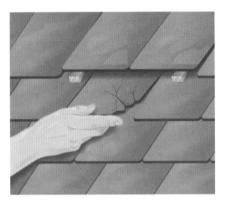

3 Fit new tile/slate

- Slide the new tile or slate into place on a builder's trowel until the two nibs on the back of the tile or slate hook on to the roof battens.
- Remove the wedges that were propping up the surrounding tiles or slates.

4 Repair flashing

- If flashing has perished, it needs to be replaced by a roofing contractor. Cracks or shrinkage, however, can be repaired relatively easily.
- If the edge of the flashing has come away from the wall, push it back into the mortar course and apply new mortar to secure it.
- If the flashing is cracked, cover it with aluminium self-adhesive flashing tape following the manufacturer's instructions.

TEMPORARY ROOF REPAIR

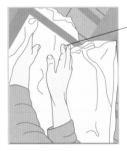

Push the plastic under the damaged area

Patch the hole
Cut a sheet of strong plastic, at least 30 cm (12 in) larger than the hole. Slide it between the roof battens and the tiles surrounding the missing or damaged tile.

Use the lower edge of the plastic sheet to drain water away from the roof

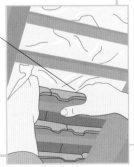

Secure sheeting
Push the lower edge of the plastic out over the lower edge of the hole, so that it directs water down the roof. Secure it with strong waterproof tape.

LEAKING GUTTERS AND DOWNPIPES

1 Check guttering and pipes

- If rainwater is overflowing from the guttering, check both the gutter and the downpipe leading from it for blockages. Obstructions are commonly caused by a build-up of leaves, or by birds' nests or balls falling into downpipes.
- If water is leaking through the guttering, check the area of the gutter that is dripping for cracks, holes, or faulty joints.
- If the guttering is not damaged, check to see if it is sagging, which prevents it from draining properly.

2 Clear blockages

- Put on protective gloves, and clear the gutter of leaves and debris so that water can flow freely.
- Clear both ends of the downpipe.
- If the blockage is caused by a bird's nest, make a hook out of a length of stiff galvanized wire. Slide the wire down one side of the nest to hook it up and out of the pipe.
- For a blockage that is out of reach, use a long, flexible rod to clear it.

! Good maintenance

- If leaves are a nuisance, fit protective mesh over the gutter and in the mouth of the downpipe. You will need to ensure that there is no build-up of leaves over the mesh, as this could cause rainwater to pour over the edge of the gutter.
- Repaint metal drains and guttering frequently to prevent them from rusting and developing holes and cracks.

3 Repair faulty guttering

- If guttering is plastic, seal a faulty joint by wrapping gutter repair tape around it. If the guttering is cracked, place the tape over the crack inside the gutter.
- Fix sagging guttering temporarily by hammering in a wooden wedge between each bracket and the gutter to hold each section in place.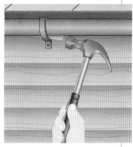
- If guttering is metal, scrape off any rust, then paint the leaking area with a sealing compound. Protect the repair until the sealant has dried, then repaint.

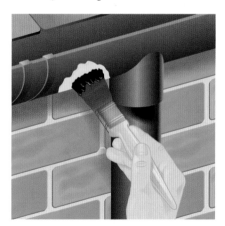

- To treat holes in metal gutters, first put on safety goggles, then wire-brush away any loose rust.
- Apply a rust-neutralizing primer, then seal small holes with a sealing compound and large holes with a special glass-fibre filler. To finish, apply black bitumen or gloss paint.

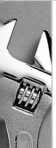

Insects and pests

As well as being a nuisance, insects can sting or bite, cockroaches, mice, and rats create unhygienic conditions, and woodworm can ruin woodwork. Take steps yourself to eliminate insects or pests or call your council or a pest controller.

FLEAS

1 Identify source

- Fleas are usually brought into the house by the family cat or dog. Make sure that all pets are regularly treated with flea killer.
- Flea eggs can lie dormant in carpets until they are activated by movement or warmth.

2 Apply flea killer

- Buy a proprietary flea repellent/ insecticide, preferably from a veterinary surgery.
- Vacuum carpets, then spray carpets and furnishings with flea killer, especially under sofas and beds.
- Treat pets and wash their bedding.

ANTS

1 Use insecticide

- Puff ant insecticide powder into the nest entrance or where the ants are entering the house.

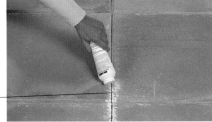

Squirt ant powder into any cracks where ants appear

2 Use jelly bait

- If the insecticide is ineffective, put down poisoned jelly bait; this will be taken back to the nest, killing the other ants.

COCKROACHES

1 Use insecticide

- If you can find where cockroaches are hiding, spray the area well with a dedicated insecticide.
- If the cockroaches remain, contact your council or a pest controller.

2 Repeat treatment

- New cockroaches are likely to appear at 4-monthly intervals; be prepared to repeat the treatment.
- Keep work surfaces clean and clear of any foodstuffs.

BEES, WASPS, AND HORNETS

1 Stay safe

- If you see a swarm of bees close to your house, get everybody inside and shut all doors and windows.
- Alert your council or the police.

2 Have nest sprayed

- If you are pestered by wasps or hornets, there is probably a nest.
- Contact your local council or ask a pest controller to spray the nest.

3 Treat stings

- Try not to antagonize bees, wasps, or hornets by spraying them with insecticide; they are more likely to sting you if they are angry.
- If you are stung, refer to p.59 for treatment. Bee stings can be removed, but wasps do not leave a sting. If you develop a minor allergic reaction, seek medical help.
- If you develop symptoms of anaphylactic shock (p.28), seek medical help immediately.

WOODWORM

1 Identify signs

- If you spot 2-mm (1/16-in) holes in furniture or structural timbers, you have woodworm. Sawdust is a sign that woodworm are active.
- Minor woodworm attacks are easy to treat (see step 2), but if an infestation is severe, you should seek professional help.

2 Treat infestation

- Brush surfaces with woodworm fluid. On furniture, use an aerosol with a nozzle to inject the fluid.
- To treat structural timbers effectively, use a large sprayer.
- To treat flooring, lift every third or fourth floorboard and spray thoroughly underneath.

MICE AND RATS

1 Block entry holes

- Small pellet-shaped droppings in your home indicate mice.
- Look for any obvious entry holes into your home and block them.

2 Put down bait

- Put down poisoned mouse bait where droppings are found. Be prepared to repeat if necessary.

3 Set traps

- Set three or four humane or spring-loaded baited mouse traps where droppings are found.
- Use peanut butter, chocolate, or cooked bacon as bait for traps.

4 Call council

- Larger droppings indicate rats; you should call your local council.

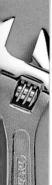

Furniture and furnishings

When accidents happen, it pays to clean up spills and stains quickly in order to avoid lasting damage to upholstered furniture and furnishings, especially carpets. Equip your home with a basic stain removal kit, see below, and you will be well-prepared to tackle even the most stubborn stains effectively.

GREASE ON CARPETS

1 Absorb grease

- Place a piece of brown paper over the mark. Put the tip of a warm iron on to the paper and press it until the grease is absorbed into the brown paper.

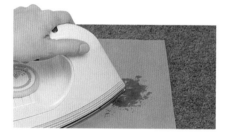

2 Use carpet cleaner

- To remove the remainder of the mark, rub carpet cleaner gently into the carpet with a sponge.

- If you have not used carpet cleaner on a particular carpet before, check for colour fastness first by testing the cleaner on carpet in an unobtrusive area.

- Wipe off the foam with a clean sponge or cloth and inspect the mark. If it you can still see a stain, or it reappears later, repeat the stain removal treatment.

GREASE ON UPHOLSTERY

1 Apply talcum powder

- Sprinkle a thick layer of talcum powder over the mark, covering it completely, and leave until the grease begins to be absorbed.

Cover grease with talcum powder

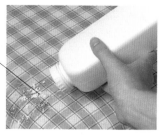

2 Brush off talcum powder

- After 10 minutes, brush off the talcum powder.
- Repeat if necessary.

ESSENTIALS

STAIN REMOVAL KIT

- Brown paper
- Talcum powder
- White kitchen towels
- Carpet cleaner
- Upholstery cleaner
- Ammonia
- Sponge
- Aerosol grease remover

GREASE ON WALLPAPER

① Blot grease

- Use white kitchen towels to blot the splash, working quickly so that the grease does not sink in.
- Hold a piece of brown paper or wallpaper against the stain.

② Use iron

- Warm a domestic iron, switch it off, then press it on to the covering paper to draw out the grease.
- Use a proprietary aerosol grease remover on any remaining traces.

RED WINE ON CARPETS

① Flush spill

- Blot the spill immediately with white kitchen towels then sponge it with warm water to flush out the stain. Pat the area dry.
- Alternatively, pour white wine on to the spill, blot up both liquids, then sponge with clear, warm water and pat dry.

Flood the red wine stain with white wine

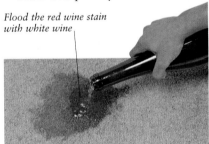

② Clean stain

- Make up some carpet cleaner then work some of the foam into the stain with a sponge, always rubbing from the edge of the stain inwards to stop it spreading.
- Sponge the stain with clear water to rinse it. Repeat the treatment until the stain has disappeared.

Rub the foam gently into the stained area

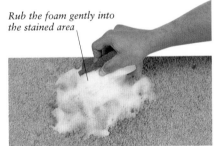

PET STAINS ON CARPETS AND UPHOLSTERY

① Remove faeces

- Wear rubber gloves.
- Scrape off the faeces with the bowl of a spoon, always scraping into the stain to avoid spreading it.
- Pour a few drops of ammonia into warm water and use the mixture to sponge the stain clean. Repeat the treatment if necessary.

② Remove urine

- Clean the stain from a carpet or upholstery using a proprietary cleaner that contains a deodorant.
- Alternatively, sponge the stain with cold water and pat dry. Follow this by sponging the stain again with cold water containing a little antiseptic.

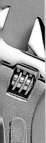

Home security

By identifying vulnerable areas of your home and taking adequate precautions, you can dramatically reduce the risk of being burgled or having your privacy invaded. Fitting additional locks and bolts is an effective way of deterring thieves. Security devices such as peepholes, security door chains, and alarms are also easy to install and not only help safeguard your property but provide peace of mind, particularly when you are away from home.

ASSESSING YOUR HOME SECURITY

1 Identify vulnerable areas

- Assess all your doors and windows for strength and security. Imagine that you have locked yourself out: which window or door would you choose to force open or break?
- Look at your house again and reassess your security.
- Contact your local crime prevention officer for advice.

2 Fit main door security devices

- Fit a five-lever mortise deadlock on the front, back, and any side doors. For added security, fit heavy bolts on the inside of each door, both top and bottom.
- Back and side doors must have sturdy locks because they are often hidden from view and badly lit, which means that a burglar can attempt entry unobserved.
- For security when answering the door, fit a strong door chain and install a peephole (p.213).
- If a door opens outwards, fit hinge bolts to the back edge (p.214) so that the door cannot be levered open on the hinge side.

3 Fit patio door locks

- Patio doors or French windows are especially vulnerable. Secure them with five-lever mortise locks as well as rack bolts (p.214), at both top and bottom, to prevent them from being forced open.

4 Fit window security devices

- Windows are popular points of entry for burglars.
- Fit window locks or rack bolts to your windows to prevent the catches being released through a smashed window. There are several types for metal and wood windows.

5 Assess lighting

- If you install security lighting to help you unlock your door on dark nights, remember that this could be equally useful to a burglar.

6 Consider an alarm

- For the best security, either buy and fit a burglar alarm yourself or have one fitted professionally.

CHOOSING LOCKS

1 Check for quality

- Always invest in good-quality locks. Cheap locks are more likely to rust and stick, which means that they are not cost-effective in the long term.
- Look for the British Standards kitemark and the number BS3621.

2 Use strong fittings

- If you fit locks in the doors and windows of your home, always use long, strong screws for maximum strength.
- If you have any doubts about your ability to fit a lock, get a locksmith to do the job for you.

FITTING A DOOR CHAIN

1 Choose chain

- Choose a strong door chain and the longest and heaviest-gauge screws possible. The chain's strength depends upon how well it is anchored to the door and frame.

Screw the fixing plates to the door and frame

2 Attach plates

- Hold the chain against the door, ideally just below the lock.
- Make pilot holes with a bradawl or drill so that both sections of the chain are aligned, then secure both fixing plates.

INSTALLING A PEEPHOLE

1 Select viewer

- Choose a telescopic viewer with as wide an angle of vision as possible. You should be able to see someone standing to the side of the door or even crouching down.
- Before you buy the peephole, make sure that the viewer is adjustable to fit any door.
- Mark the best position for the peephole, ideally in the centre of the door at eye level.

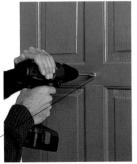

Drill the hole for the peephole at eye level

2 Fit peephole

- Using the correct-sized drill bit, usually 12 mm (½ in), drill a hole right through the door.
- Insert the barrel of the viewer into the hole from the outside and screw on the eyepiece from the inside.
- Check that the lighting outside your front door is sufficiently bright for you to be able to see out clearly at night.

FITTING HINGE BOLTS

1 Position bolts

- Wedge the door fully open and mark the centre of the hinge edge of the door about 75 mm (3 in) in from both hinges.
- Drill holes at the marked points to the width and depth specified by the manufacturer.
- Fit the bolts into the holes and partially close the door so that the bolts mark the door frame.

Insert the bolts into the drilled holes

2 Fit cover plates

- At the marked points, drill holes into the door frame to the width and depth of the protruding bolts, allowing a little more for clearance.
- Close the door to check that it shuts easily. Enlarge the width or depth of the holes as necessary.
- Open the door and hold cover plates over the holes. Mark the edge of each plate with a pencil.
- Chisel out the recesses so that the plates lie flush with the cover frame.
- Screw the plates in place.

FITTING A RACK BOLT

1 Drill holes for barrel and key

- Mark a central point on the front edge of the door where you want to fit the bolt.
- Drill a hole at the marked point to the width and depth given on the manufacturer's instructions.

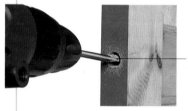

Drill into the opening edge of the door

- Use a try square to mark a line transferring the centre of the hole to the inside face of the door.
- Mark the keyhole, then drill a hole (see manufacturer's instructions for width and depth) through the inside face of the door only.

2 Fit bolt and plate

- Screw the keyhole plate to the door.
- Insert the bolt into the hole then draw round the faceplate to mark its recess. Pare out the wood with a chisel. Screw the bolt to the door.
- Insert the key and turn the bolt to mark the door frame, then drill a hole to a depth that matches the length of the bolt.
- Fit the locking plate over the hole.

Mark the shape of the faceplate recess

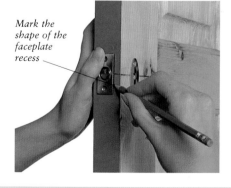

JAMMED LOCK

1 Add lubricant

- If a lock is jammed, do not try to force the key to turn: you could break the key in the lock.
- Add a little dry lubricant, such as graphite powder, into the lock, or apply a few drops of easing oil to lubricate the key.

2 Work key

- Work the key gently in and out of the lock, adding a little more lubricant if necessary.
- If this fails, either replace the cylinder if it is a cylinder lock (see below) or replace the lock body of a mortise lock (see below).

JAMMED CYLINDER LOCK

1 Remove cylinder

- If a cylinder lock is jammed (see above) or if you are worried about the security of your existing lock, replace the cylinder.
- Unscrew the lock body on the internal side of the door, then unscrew the cylinder.
- Remove the cylinder from its cavity by pulling it from the external side of the door.

Slide the new cylinder into the existing cylinder hole

2 Fit new cylinder

- Insert a new cylinder by sliding it into the cylinder hole and screwing it into place.
- Put the lock body back in position and refix the holding screws.

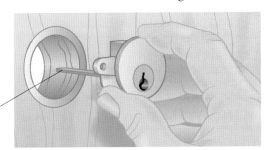

DAMAGED MORTISE LOCK

1 Replace striking plate

- If a striking plate is damaged, causing a door to stick as it closes, buy a replacement.
- Unscrew the damaged striking plate from its position in the door jamb.
- Insert a replacement striking plate in exactly the same position and screw it into place.

2 Replace lock body

- If a mortise lock is jammed (see above) or if you are worried about the security of your existing lock, replace the lock body.
- Unscrew the lock body and remove it from its mortise in the door.
- Insert a replacement lock body into the mortise and screw it into place. If the fit is too tight, use a wood chisel to enlarge the recess slightly.

DEALING WITH INTRUDERS

1 Be vigilant

- If you arrive home and see anyone loitering outside, pass by your house and ask a neighbour to accompany you to the door.
- If you return home to find that the front door is open, do not enter your home. Move a safe distance away and, if you have a mobile phone, call the police. Alternatively, go to a neighbour and phone the police from there.
- If you come home and your key won't open the door, it could mean that an intruder has secured the door from inside so as not to be disturbed. Move away quickly and phone the police.
- If you return home to find that your home has been ransacked, call the police immediately. Do not touch anything until the police arrive in case you destroy any fingerprints left by burglars.

2 Make a noise

- If you do enter your home and meet an intruder, run out and shout or scream as loudly as you can.
- Don't try to apprehend him or her.

3 Stay calm

- If you must face the intruder, keep calm and try not to provoke a reaction by making threats.
- Try to memorize as much as you can of the intruder's appearance, mannerisms, and speech so that you can provide the police with an accurate description.

4 Call the police

- Dial 999 or telephone your local police station.
- Try to give the police as much information as possible.

DEALING WITH A NIGHT INTRUDER

- If you are woken in the night by unusual noises or the sound of breaking glass, phone the police.
- Keep your mobile phone by the bed and switched on so that you can still call for help if the telephone line has been cut.
- If you are alone in the house, talk loudly as if you have a companion in the room. You could also switch on the lights and make a lot of noise. Most intruders will leave as soon as they hear noise.
- Do not go downstairs to investigate.

- Do not keep an offensive weapon with a view to defending your property. No items, however valuable, are worth serious injury or even death.
- If you meet the intruder, stay calm and try to memorize his or her appearance.

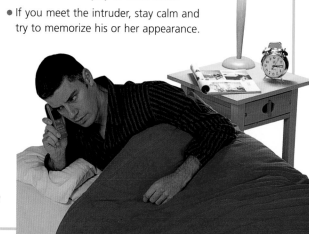

Responding to a disturbance
When you phone the police, you will be advised on whether to make a noise or to pretend that you are asleep. Stay in bed until the police arrive.

COPING AFTER A BREAK-IN

1 Don't move anything

- If you discover that your home has been broken into, try to keep calm.
- Do not touch anything. The police will want to check the crime scene and look for fingerprints.

2 Call police

- Dial 999 or telephone your local police station.
- When the police arrive, they will talk to you about the burglary, ask what has been taken, then take a statement. They will then provide you with a crime reference number for your insurance company.

3 List missing items

- Start to make a list of what you think has been taken. This process can go on for days, because many items will be missed only when you come to try to use or find them. The police should supply you with a form for your list.
- Give as clear a description as you can of all items, and provide photographs of valuables, if you have them.
- Indicate on the list which, if any, items have been security marked.

4 Secure premises

- If burglars have forced entry by smashing glass, make a temporary repair for security (p.200).
- Assess how the burglar(s) gained access to your home and take steps to make it more secure by installing additional locks or bolts (p.214).

5 Contact insurers

- Contact your insurance company and explain what has happened.
- The insurance company and/or loss adjuster will require the crime reference number and a detailed list of what has been stolen.

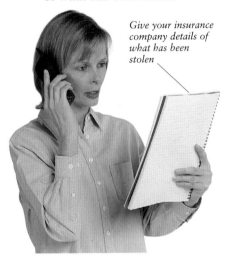

Give your insurance company details of what has been stolen

6 Keep in contact with police

- If you move house while the investigation is still ongoing, notify the police of your new address.
- If you discover more items missing or damage caused, contact the officer handling your case as well as your insurance company.

SEEKING ADVICE

- If you are the victim of a burglary or assault, you will be contacted by Victim Support, an organization that provides counselling and help for victims of crime.
- Talk to friends and family about your experience. They may be able to offer you reassurance and comfort.

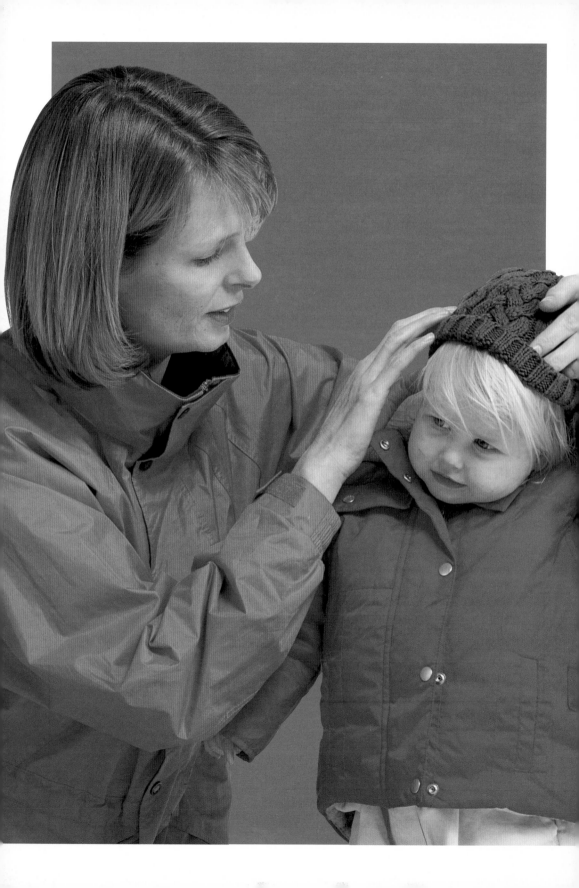

4
NATURAL
DISASTERS

Surviving any kind of natural disaster depends largely on being prepared. If you know how to protect your home and family, what the early warnings mean, and how to evacuate if you are advised to do so, you will be ready for most disaster situations. Once a disaster is over, life may not return to normal for some time, so you also need to know how to cope with power cuts, damage to your home, and possible water shortages. If evacuated, you may even have to survive outside for a while until help arrives.

Planning for disaster

If you live in an area that is at risk from certain types of natural disaster, planning and preparing for an emergency will help protect you and your family should the worst happen. Take steps to safeguard your home and garden and choose a safe place inside to shelter. If hurricanes are a threat, find out where your local shelter is, and assemble essential equipment that may help you survive the aftermath.

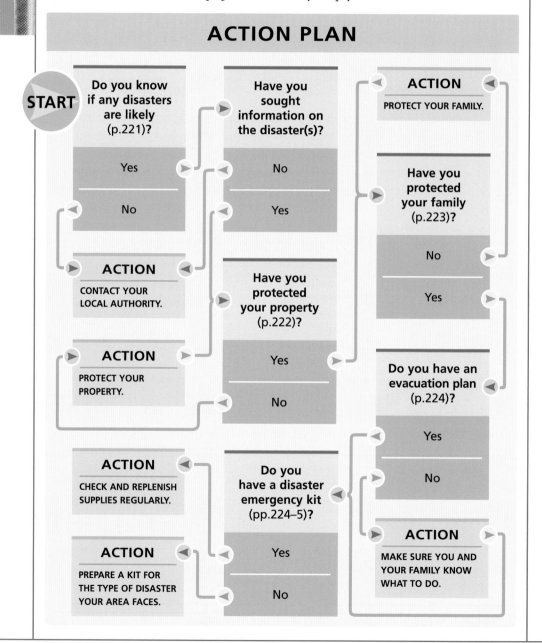

ACTION PLAN

START

Do you know if any disasters are likely (p.221)?

Yes

No

ACTION

CONTACT YOUR LOCAL AUTHORITY.

ACTION

PROTECT YOUR PROPERTY.

ACTION

CHECK AND REPLENISH SUPPLIES REGULARLY.

ACTION

PREPARE A KIT FOR THE TYPE OF DISASTER YOUR AREA FACES.

Have you sought information on the disaster(s)?

No

Yes

Have you protected your property (p.222)?

Yes

No

Do you have a disaster emergency kit (pp.224–5)?

Yes

No

ACTION

PROTECT YOUR FAMILY.

Have you protected your family (p.223)?

No

Yes

Do you have an evacuation plan (p.224)?

Yes

No

ACTION

MAKE SURE YOU AND YOUR FAMILY KNOW WHAT TO DO.

ASSESSING YOUR RISK

- Volcanic eruptions and earthquakes occur around geological fault lines and can both produce tsunamis.

- Hurricanes mostly affect areas around the Atlantic basin and the Pacific basin, where they are known as tropical cyclones. They are often accompanied by tornadoes.

- Flooding can occur almost anywhere, although the most serious floods are usually caused by very high tides.

- Wildfires occur in many countries – 80 per cent are started by humans.

- Extreme cold occurs in much of the northern hemisphere but many countries experience freezes in winter.

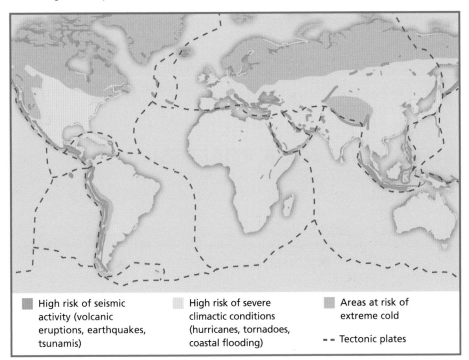

High risk of seismic activity (volcanic eruptions, earthquakes, tsunamis)	High risk of severe climactic conditions (hurricanes, tornadoes, coastal flooding)	Areas at risk of extreme cold
		- - Tectonic plates

1 Be informed

- Contact your local authority to find out whether your area is prone to any specific types of disaster. Ask for information about each type.

- If your area is prone to flooding, contact your local authority to find the height at which a flood would affect your home.

- Before travelling abroad or moving some distance to a new home, find out about disaster risks in that area.

- Learn about the possible effects of disasters that may strike your area.

2 Reduce risk

- Take steps now to protect your property against natural disasters. Your home will be less vulnerable to disaster if you take sensible precautions and carry out routine building maintenance (p.222).

- Protect your family by coming up with a family disaster plan (p.223) and making sure that you are all prepared for evacuation (p.224).

- Always keep abreast of the weather situation and local plans regarding shelters and evacuation.

PROTECTING YOUR HOME

- Arrange for unsafe or old chimney stacks to be removed or repointed.
- Replace cracked or broken slates or tiles on the roof (p.206). Check that roof flashings are watertight. If any are loose or damaged, have them repaired or replaced (p.206).
- Keep gutters and downpipes clear and in good repair (p.207).
- If you live in an area at risk from tornadoes or hurricanes, fit special hurricane shutters as a precaution.
- Alternatively, fix wooden frames to the windows so that you can board them up quickly (p.234).

- Check and, if necessary, repair any obvious weaknesses in the structure of your house, such as cracks that are wider than 3 mm (⅛ in).
- If your area is at risk from flooding, make sure that you have sufficient sandbags to block all potential water entry points, such as external doors, airbricks, and vents (p.228).
- Ensure that any adults know how to turn off gas, electricity, and water at the mains, in case you need to do this in a hurry before leaving.
- Check that you have adequate insurance cover for disasters that are likely to strike in your area.

PROTECTING YOUR POSSESSIONS

- Make sure that shelves are securely fastened to the wall.
- Keep heavier items on lower shelves so that if a disaster occurs and they fall, they are far less likely to cause someone a serious injury.
- If flooding is a risk in your area, keep very precious items on higher shelves to protect them from water damage. Alternatively, move your most valuable possessions upstairs.

- Bolt any tall pieces of furniture, boilers, and other heavy items to the wall or floor (p.238) to ensure that they are stable and secure.
- Add additional fittings to secure heavy light fixtures to ceilings.
- Keep a supply of housebricks that you can use to raise heavy furniture out of reach of flood water.
- Keep a fire extinguisher and blanket to put out minor house fires.

PROTECTING YOUR GARDEN

- Remove any diseased or broken tree branches that could be blown about by high winds. Thin out crowded branches to reduce wind resistance.
- If you live in an area that is prone to wildfire, create a safety zone around your home (p.232).
- During hurricane/tornado seasons, bring indoors any garden furniture or children's play equipment that is not anchored to the ground, or move it into a garage.

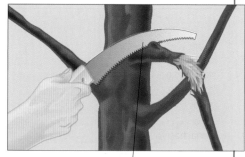

Cut off any broken branches before high winds rip them off

PROTECTING YOUR FAMILY

1 Be informed

- Contact your local authority to find out if whether any warning signals will be issued and what action you should take (see box below).
- If you live in an area that is prone to certain disasters, you may be issued with a telephone number to ring for up-to-date information and warnings. You may also find advice on the Internet (see pp.250–251 for recommended websites).
- Prior to a disaster, public address systems such as loudhailers may be used to inform people quickly, and provide instructions on what to do.
- If you are likely to be evacuated to an emergency shelter, find out now where the nearest shelters are and how you will get to them.

2 Think ahead

- Keep emergency contact numbers near the telephone and ensure that everyone knows where they are.
- Consider how to help the elderly and physically disabled.
- Plan how you are going to look after any pets. Keep pet carriers for small family pets if necessary.
- Assemble essential items that you will need if disaster strikes (p.225).

3 Make a family disaster plan

- Discuss how to prepare for disaster.
- Make sure that children understand the dangers of severe weather and any other disasters that are likely to threaten your area.
- Some natural disasters, including lightning strikes, earthquakes, and volcanic eruptions, can cause house fires; agree on a meeting place just outside the home so that you can check that everyone is safely out of the building in the event of a fire.
- Arrange a second meeting place some distance away, such as at a friend's or relative's home, should you have to leave the immediate area. Make sure that everyone has the address and telephone number.
- Choose at least two escape routes from your home and each room.
- Identify safe places in your home where you could shelter if you are advised to stay indoors or if you do not have time to leave before a disaster strikes.
- Plan what the family needs to do in an evacuation (p.224).
- Discuss how to make contact and reunite family members should a disaster occur when you are not all at home together.

UNDERSTANDING EARLY WARNINGS

- If you live in a hurricane or tornado zone, be prepared for a "watch" (possible disaster) and then a "warning" (probable or imminent disaster) as the hurricane or tornado approaches your area.
- If you live in a tsunami area, an "advisory" is the first alert, followed by a "watch" (possible) and "warning" (imminent).
- If you live in an area at risk from flooding, a "watch" (possible) may be followed by a "warning" (imminent) and then a "severe warning" (imminent and severe).
- In areas of particular risk, there may be a system for sending warning messages directly to people at home or at work by telephone, fax, or pager, if their homes are threatened.

EVACUATING SAFELY

1 Follow instructions

- Prepare to evacuate if you are told to do so by your local authority or the emergency services, or if you feel in danger in your own home.
- Follow any evacuation instructions carefully: there may be limits on what you can take with you.

2 Gather family members

- Assemble family members quickly, collect your disaster emergency kit (p.225), and decide whether you should leave by car or go on foot.
- Help the elderly and children to evacuate. Having to leave home in a disaster situation will be distressing, so remain calm and be reassuring.
- Think how to help disabled people evacuate; for example, you may need to accommodate a wheelchair.
- Put small pets into pet carriers; take dogs with you in the car or put them on leads if you leave on foot.

3 Take precautions

- If high winds are forecast, bring children's play equipment and garden furniture indoors (p.222).
- Call the friend/relative whom you agreed in your disaster plan should be your second point of contact. Explain where you are going.
- Use telephones and mobile phones only if it is essential to get in touch with family or friends – otherwise keep lines free for emergency calls.
- Always turn off the gas, electricity, and water before leaving.
- Close and lock all your external doors and windows as you leave, including doors to outbuildings.

4 Be a good neighbour

- Make sure that your neighbours are aware of the need to evacuate.
- Go the the aid of elderly or disabled neighbours who may be unable to evacuate without your assistance.

PREPARING A DISASTER EMERGENCY KIT

1 Organize basic items

- List the items you would need to take with you if advised to evacuate (see p.225 for suggestions).
- The amount of equipment you will need depends on the type and extent of disaster likely to affect your area.
- Assemble these items.
- Encourage your children to help with the planning and packing of your family emergency kit.

2 Consider extras

- If you live in an area that is at risk of a major disaster, you may well have to survive outside for several days. Plan to take water-purifying tablets. Keep a plastic bucket with lid and bin liners (to be used as a toilet) and toilet rolls.
- If you live near a volcano, add a disposable dust mask and goggles for each family member.
- If you have a small pet, keep a pet carrier suitable for carrying it.

3 Keep kit ready

- Keep your disaster emergency kit in a safe accessible place, such as in the garage, and ensure that all family members know where it is.
- Practise evacuating your home, loading the kit into the car, and leaving as quickly as possible.
- Replace your water supplies every 6 months and make regular checks on sell-by dates of all foods.
- Test batteries at regular intervals.
- Note the expiry dates on first-aid and prescription medicines and replace any that are out of date.

4 Assess situation

- If evacuating by car, you should be able to load your kit into the boot.
- If evacuating on foot, decide how much kit you can carry by sharing the load among family members.
- In the case of a mass evacuation, emergency shelter will be provided in local community buildings. In such situations you do not need to take food, water, or bedding.
- In situations where it may be some time before you can return home, take plenty of clothing and toys or games to occupy children.

DISASTER EMERGENCY KIT

MEDICAL EQUIPMENT
Pack a first-aid kit and any over-the-counter or prescription medicines needed

TORCHES AND BATTERIES
Ideally, have one torch per family member, plus plenty of spare batteries

CANDLES AND MATCHES
These are for back-up lighting should there be a prolonged power cut

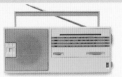

BATTERY-POWERED RADIO
Use this for news of the disaster and local authority instructions

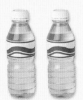

WATER
Store 4.5 litres (8 pints) of water per person per day

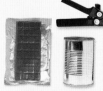

FOOD AND CAN OPENER
Store enough canned or dried food for 3 days per person

FAMILY DOCUMENTS
Keep passports and family documents in a waterproof wallet with emergency money

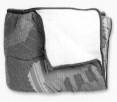

BEDDING
Allow one sleeping bag or blanket per person for sleeping outside

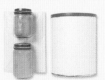

BABY FOOD AND MILK
Take jars, cans, and a spoon, formula mixes, and bottles

NAPPIES AND CREAMS
Keep supplies of disposable nappies and nappy cream

SHOES AND CLOTHES
Allow a change of footwear and clothing per person

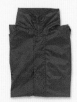

RAINWEAR
Keep a lightweight waterproof for each family member

Severe storm

► For FLOOD see p.228

High winds during a severe storm can cause damage to roofing, chimneys, and windows, while heavy rain can result in leaks and flooding. But there are steps you can take to protect against, and cope with, storm damage. Lightning can also be dangerous if you are out in the open, so make sure that you know what to do.

COPING WITH A SEVERE STORM

1 Take precautions

- Stay inside during the storm.
- Fasten doors and windows tightly and check that doors to garden sheds and garages are also shut.
- Keep torches, candles, and matches ready in case of power cuts.
- If a thunderstorm is on the way, disconnect television aerials from their sockets and unplug computers and televisions. Power surges from lightning can start fires and cause considerable damage.
- Have a couple of buckets ready so that you can place them underneath leaks if the roof is damaged.
- Put away garden furniture.

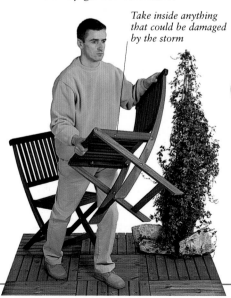

Take inside anything that could be damaged by the storm

2 Deal with leaks

- If water starts dripping through the ceiling, it probably means that the roof is damaged or that flashing has worked loose, in which case water will seep through it.
- Place buckets under the drips and go into the roof to look for a leak.
- If a roof tile or slate is damaged or missing, make a temporary repair with plastic sheeting (p.206).
- If water is coming in around the chimney stack, repair or replace flashing after the storm (p.206).
- If water is pooling outside your house, use a stiff broom to sweep it away downhill.
- If the water continues to rise, block all gaps under and around doors with sandbags (p.228).

3 Minimize damage

- If a window is blown in, move anything valuable out of the room. Block the window with boarding, nailing it from the inside, or move a large piece of furniture, such as a wardrobe, in front of it.
- If a chimney stack is blown off, water may find its way down the chimney. Use boards to block all fireplaces and so prevent any rubble from coming down into the room.

OUTSIDE IN LIGHTNING

① Get to safety

- If you are out in a storm and see lightning approaching, look for shelter in a low area, such as in a ditch or on the side of a hill, away from tall trees and poles, and water.
- Remember that any thunderstorm may produce lightning.
- Keep well away from metal objects, such as fences or pylons: these can pose a particular danger because a lightning spark will arc off metal, striking anyone standing nearby.
- If you are riding a bicycle, get off, leave the bicycle, and take shelter.
- If you are riding a horse, get off, tether the horse safely to whatever is available, then shelter.
- If you are in a car with a metal roof, stay where you are: the metal shell will protect you and the lightning will earth itself through the rubber wheels.
- If you are out in a boat, head for land immediately.

DO'S AND DON'TS

DO	DON'T
• Get on to open land.	• Stand on high ground, such as on top of a hill.
• Stay away from tall trees or rocks.	• Think that you are protected by wearing rubber-soled shoes or wellington boots.
• Make yourself as small and as low as you can.	
• Protect your head from a possible strike.	• Kneel or sit down on wet material.
• Stay in your car if you are out driving.	• Carry metal objects.

② Protect yourself

- Do not carry anything with a metal rod that might conduct lightning, such as umbrellas or golf clubs.
- If you feel your hair stand on end, lightning is about to strike.
- If you are near trees or rocks, run for open ground, if you have time. If not, kneel down, bend forwards to protect your head, and put your hands on your knees.
  - If you are on open ground, crouch down.
    - It is important to protect your head, which is the most vulnerable part of your body, and to minimize contact with the ground.

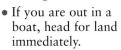

Keep your head lower than the rest of your body

! If someone is struck by lightning

- A bolt of lightning can be fatal if it strikes someone on the head and then travels down to the ground. It can also cause severe burns, broken bones, and cuts; it can render a person unconscious; and it can set clothing on fire.
- Do not touch someone who has been struck by lightning if he or she is either very wet or is in water; you could be electrocuted. This is because the electrical discharge will not have dispersed and is still within the body.

- If the person's clothing is on fire, follow the instructions on p.182.
- Call an ambulance immediately, even if the person appears to be unharmed.
- Treat the burns (pp.48–9).
- If the person is not breathing, start rescue breathing (pp.16–17).
- If the person has no signs of circulation, start CPR (pp.18–20).

Flood

◀ For SEVERE STORM see p.226 ▶ For TSUNAMI see p.242

Heavy rainfall, snow melt, rivers changing course, dams collapsing, and high tides in coastal areas can all cause floods. If you live in an area prone to flooding, recognize the difference between a "flood watch" (flooding is possible), a "flood warning" (flooding is expected), and a "severe flood warning" (severe flooding is expected), and take the necessary measures to protect your family and home.

PREPARING FOR A FLOOD

① Plan ahead

- Contact your local council to find out at what height flooding will affect your home.
- Listen for the early flood warnings issued by weather forecasters and the Environment Agency.
- Buy enough house bricks to enable you to raise wooden or upholstered furniture off the floor and out of the flood water.
- Buy sandbags and sand if water is likely to rise above door level.
- Keep your important documents in plastic wallets in a safe place.

② Prepare home

- Block all airbricks and gaps under and around external doors with sandbags (see box below).
- If flood water is forecast to rise up to window height, place sandbags along external window sills too.
- Take up your carpets and carry them upstairs for safety, with all the valuables that you can move.
- Fill clean baths, sinks, and plastic bottles with cold water.
- Turn off electricity and gas supplies; flooded wiring can cause fires.
- Use bricks to raise furniture.

PROTECTING YOUR HOME WITH SANDBAGS

- Use sandbags to seal entry points around doors as well as airbricks and vents. Also seal windows if the water is likely to rise that high.
- Half-fill the sandbag casings with sand. If you run out of casings, make your own from plastic carrier bags, pillow cases, or even tights.
- Place the first row of bags in position, butting them up against each other, end to end, and then stamp down on them to mould the ends together.
- Lay the second row on top, staggering the bags, and stamping down on them to mould them into the row below. This will prevent seepage through gaps.
- If your wall needs to be three or four rows tall, lay two rows side by side, followed by a second double row, then one or more single rows on top.

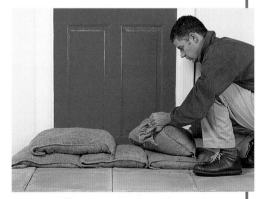

Using sandbags
Lay the second row of bags in place, staggering the bags over the first row in a brickwork-like formation.

SURVIVING A FLOOD

1 Stay inside

- If you can, move upstairs, taking with you food, water, and other emergency supplies, pets, plus any valuables and important papers.

Take plenty of water with you

Take small pets upstairs with you in pet carriers

If your child is upset by the flood, carry her to safety

- If flood water rises quickly, leaving you no time to move your valuables upstairs, put them on high shelves to keep them out of the water.
- Be aware that flood water can weaken structural foundations causing buildings to sink; floors may crack and, in severe cases, walls may even collapse. Regularly check for cracks in what you can see of your walls, floors, doors, staircases, and windows.
- Listen to your radio for updated local information and follow any official instructions.
- Observe water levels outside to see how fast they are rising.
- Use your supplies of drinking water until you are told that the mains water is not contaminated.

2 Evacuation

- If you are told to evacuate, follow the instructions carefully.
- In addition to taking your disaster emergency kit (p.225), take all the clothing you can. It may be days or, in some situations, weeks before you are able to return home.

3 Signal for help

- If the water has risen to the point that you are unable to leave safely on foot, or you feel that your life is in danger if you stay where you are, you need to signal for help.
- Lean out of an upstairs window or climb on to the roof and signal your distress by shouting and/or waving something bright.

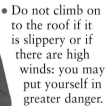

- Do not climb on to the roof if it is slippery or if there are high winds: you may put yourself in greater danger.

Attract attention by shouting and waving

! If you are outside

- Be very careful when walking through flood water: just 15 cm (6 in) of fast-flowing water can unbalance you and cause you to fall.
- If possible, use a stick to feel the ground before you step on it: hazards hidden under the water could be highly dangerous.
- Avoid riverbanks or sea defences, which could collapse, and beware of large waves.
- Minimize contact with flood water: it could be contaminated with sewage.

Extreme cold

Heavy snowfall and very low temperatures can produce difficult conditions both at home and outside, especially if cold weather continues for a long period. Prepare for wintry conditions well in advance by checking that your house is well-insulated in summer or early autumn. During a freeze, keep warm and stay safe, preferably indoors, and be a good neighbour to the elderly or frail.

PREPARING FOR EXTREME COLD

1 Check insulation

- Fix self-adhesive foam strips around loose-fitting doors and windows; this will help prevent draughts.
- Fit draught excluders across the bottoms of external doors.
- Hang a heavy curtain at the front door to keep the hall draught-free.
- To improve insulation, fix sheets of glass in frames across single glazed windows. You can also use a special heat-sensitive plastic film as a temporary measure (see box right), which is cheaper, but less efficient.
- Check that outdoor pipes and taps are properly insulated.
- Check that the attic, and any pipes and water tanks within it, are well insulated. However, do not place insulation under a cold water tank, because this will prevent warmth rising from rooms below.

2 Check heating

- Turn on your central heating for a trial run to check that it is working efficiently. If you discover problems see p.193 for advice.
- Stick aluminium foil sheets, shiny side out, behind radiators to reflect heat back into the room. This is particularly important for any radiators against external walls.

3 Take precautions

- Buy low-wattage electric heaters that you can leave on overnight to keep rooms above freezing point.
- If you depend on electricity, buy a portable gas heater so that you will be able to keep warm if power lines should come down.
- If you have a wood or coal fire, stock up on fuel and matches.
- Maintain supplies of medicines.
- If your cooker is electric, stock up on foods that do not need cooking.

TEMPORARY INSULATION

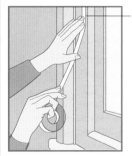

Stick lengths of tape in place

Apply adhesive tape
Put lengths of double-sided adhesive tape down the sides and across the top and bottom of the window. Allow adhesive to harden for 1 hour.

Keep the hairdryer moving to smooth film

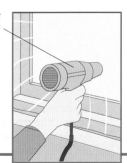

Stretch plastic
Press heat-sensitive plastic film across the window and on to the adhesive strips. Hold a hairdryer a few centimetres away and warm the plastic until the film is quite taut.

SURVIVING EXTREME COLD

1 Stay warm

- Keep the heating on day and night at a low setting so that your home does not become cold and water pipes do not freeze. Alternatively, use low-wattage electric heaters.
- If you are worried about costly fuel bills, heat only the rooms that you need to use, and close the doors to unheated rooms.
- Close the curtains to keep the heat in, but air rooms daily so that they do not become stuffy.

2 Stay inside

- When conditions are icy, do not venture outside unless it is essential. If you must go out, see the box on the right for sensible advice.
- Avoid driving unless your journey is absolutely necessary. If you will be travelling through rural or hilly terrain, go prepared to be caught in a snowdrift or blizzard (see below).
- Check that you have a cold-weather kit in your car (see box right) in case of emergencies.
- Always take a mobile phone, whether you are on foot or in a car.
- If you live in an avalanche area and an avalanche warning is issued, stay inside unless told to evacuate.

IF YOU HAVE TO GO OUT

- Dress warmly in layers of light clothing, a jacket or coat, hat, scarf, and gloves.
- Wear sturdy boots with a deep tread and be careful to take small, firm steps; point your toes inwards on downhill slopes and bend your knees slightly if the going is steep.
- Be careful on icy surfaces; try to find something to hold on to, such as a railing.
- Be particularly careful if you are elderly: your more brittle bones may fracture more easily.

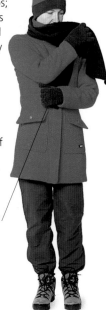

Cover your hands and head

Preventing heat loss
A hat is the most important item of clothing, because most body heat is lost through the head

ESSENTIALS

COLD-WEATHER CAR KIT

- Shovel
- Blankets and coats
- Grit or sacking
- Torch and batteries
- High-energy food
- Water

! If your car gets stuck in snow

- Drive very slowly backwards and forwards, moving only slightly each time, until your car can gradually make a track for itself.
- If this does not work, use a shovel to clear away snow from around the wheels, then put down grit or sacking to give the tyres something to grip. Drive forwards very slowly. Once the car is clear of the snow, do not stop until you have reached safety.

- If you are unable to move the car, do not try to walk to safety: stay inside the vehicle.
- Wrap yourself in blankets or newspaper.
- Turn on the engine and run the heater for 10 minutes every hour to conserve petrol.
- Open a window occasionally to let in air.
- Try to stay awake; the risk of hypothermia (p.54) is greater if you fall asleep.

Wildfire

Most forest fires, which includes fires in woodland, forest, heath, and moorland, and bushfires, occur in hot, dry weather. These fires can spread rapidly to cover vast areas and, once they have taken hold, are very difficult to control. Protect your home against wildfire by creating a safety zone, take sensible precautions to safeguard your family, and know what to do if wildfire threatens your home.

PROTECTING AGAINST WILDFIRE

1 Create a safe zone

- Remove all flammable vegetation, dead branches, leaves, and twigs, and mow grass within 9 m (30 ft) of your home (30 m/100 ft if you live in a pine forest).
- Keep this zone clear to ensure that any wildfire will find little to burn and pass by your house.
- Consider felling trees inside the zone other than fire-resistant hardwoods such as oak, beech, or ash.
- Store flammable items, such as old newspapers, supplies of firewood, and wooden garden furniture, well outside the safety zone.

2 Be prepared

- Install a garden hose that is long enough to reach the full extent of your house and garden.
- Keep any tools that could be used to beat out fire, such as brushes and spades, in a handy, safe place.
- Plan several escape routes away from your home by car and by foot.
- Arrange to stay elsewhere in case you have to evacuate the area.
- Keep plenty of fuel in your car so that you can escape quickly in the event of an emergency.
- Make sure that gutters and drains are clear of debris (p.207).

SURVIVING WILDFIRE

1 Be ready to evacuate

- If a wildfire appears to be heading in your direction, check that your car has ample fuel, then park it facing your main route of escape.
- Place your disaster emergency kit (p.225) in the boot, then close all the doors and windows and leave your key in the ignition.
- Assemble your pets and fire tools (see Be prepared, above).

2 Protect your home

- Bring wooden garden furniture inside the house, if necessary.
- Use your garden hose to soak both the safety zone and the house.
- Close all the windows, doors, and air vents. Draw heavy curtains, pull down blinds, and take down any lightweight curtains.
- Move flammable furniture into the centre of the house, away from any windows and glass doors.

3 Get to safety

- Keep the radio on and listen out for updated local information and official instructions.
- If you are told to evacuate, follow the instructions carefully.

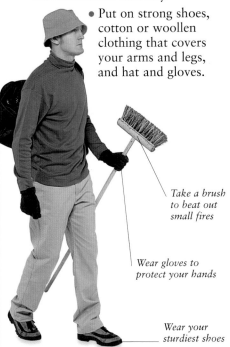

- Put on strong shoes, cotton or woollen clothing that covers your arms and legs, and hat and gloves.

Take a brush to beat out small fires

Wear gloves to protect your hands

Wear your sturdiest shoes

- Take your pets, disaster emergency kit, and fire tools with you.
- Choose a planned route that will take you away from the fire, but keep alert for any alterations in its speed and direction.

4 Use your car as protection

- If you are overtaken by flames in the car, stay inside your vehicle. You are safer inside your car than outside in the thick smoke and fierce heat, even with the risk that the fuel tank may explode.
- Explain to any passengers the risks of leaving the car.

5 Follow official instructions

- Do not return home until you have been given the all-clear.
- When you are allowed to return home, proceed with caution – small fires may still be blazing.
- As a precaution against further fires, re-soak your house and the entire safety zone with water.
- If your house has been damaged by fire, check with the fire service that it is safe to enter the building.
- Arrange temporary accommodation if necessary.
- If the fire has passed by your house, check for any smoke damage that may require an insurance claim. Take photographs, if you can, to support any future claim.

! If you are outside

- Try to run diagonally away from the fire to get out of its path. Aim for an open area, a road, or a river, if possible. If the fire comes close, lay down, curl into a ball, and cover your head, hands, and as much of your body as possible with a jacket.
- If your clothing catches fire, quickly smother the flames with a coat and then roll around on the ground to extinguish them (p.182).

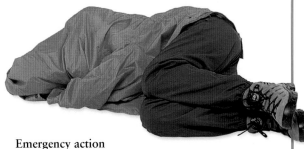

Emergency action
If fire is blocking all your escape routes, head for a dip or hollow and roll into a ball.

Hurricane

◀ For **FLOOD** see p.228 ▶ For **TORNADO** see p.236

Hurricanes are extremely violent storms, producing strong winds of up to 305 km/h (190 mph) and torrential rain. Tornadoes may occur simultaneously or in the hurricane's wake. Flooding may also follow. Many hurricanes can be predicted, enabling people to protect their homes and evacuate their families in good time. If you live in an area that is prone to hurricanes, make sure that you know the difference between a "hurricane watch" (a hurricane is possible within 36 hours) and a "hurricane warning" (a hurricane is likely within 24 hours).

PREPARING FOR A HURRICANE

1 Plan ahead

- Install hurricane shutters or buy sheets of plywood and strips of wood for boarding windows (see box below). Nail the frames in position and prepare the plywood sheets for fitting when necessary.
- Find out which hurricane shelter is closest to your home.

2 Take precautions

- Keep alert for a "hurricane watch" and listen to local radio stations for updates on the situation.
- If a "hurricane watch" turns into a "hurricane warning", make final preparations to your home.
- Choose a safe part of the house where family members can gather. The ideal place is a room in the centre of the house that does not have windows (such as a hallway).
- Close the hurricane shutters or fix boards in place (see box right).
- Secure external and garage doors.
- Fill clean baths, sinks, containers, and plastic bottles with water to ensure an uncontaminated supply.

3 Get to safety

- If you live in a mobile home, leave immediately and head towards open ground or a hurricane shelter.
- If you live in a house and you are advised to evacuate, follow all the instructions carefully.
- Avoid coastal and river roads on your way to a hurricane shelter – these routes may be flooded.

BOARDING WINDOWS

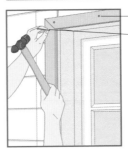

Predrill screw holes

Secure frame in place

Make outer frame
Cut strips of wood to fit around the outside of the window frame. Predrill with holes 15 cm (6 in) apart. Nail the strips in place to form a frame.

Screw board in place

Align screw holes

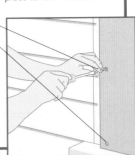

Attach cover
Cut sheets of 1-cm (½-in) plywood to fit window frame. Predrill holes to align with the frame. Screw cover in place.

DURING A HURRICANE

1 Stay informed

- Keep your radio on and listen for updated local information or any official instructions. You may be asked to turn off utilities or to evacuate at any point.
- If you are advised to evacuate, follow all the instructions carefully.

2 Stay indoors

- Do not evacuate unless advised to do so, or you feel that it would endanger life to remain at home.
- Close all interior doors and place doorstops under them.
- Close all curtains and blinds.
- Turn off major appliances if advised to do so, or if power fails.
- Make sure that all household pets are inside and keep them in pet carriers with adequate water.
- Go to your chosen safe place and stay under a table, if there is one.
- If you feel that the house is starting to collapse around you, try to move quickly under a sturdy bed or a pile of mattresses; if there is no time to move, stay under the table.

3 Stay safe

- Be aware that when the eye of the storm passes overhead, it may appear that a hurricane is over. However, winds will start blowing again from the opposite direction within the hour, and this can often be the worst part of the storm.
- Listen for warnings of tornadoes (p.236) or severe flooding (p.228), both of which often occur in the aftermath of a hurricane.
- Stay where you are until you are sure that the hurricane has passed.

! If you are outside

- Lie flat on the ground and crawl on your stomach to find shelter, such as an outcrop of rock, a ditch, or a low wall.
- Cover your head with your hands or a coat.
- Do not shelter too close to trees because branches may break off or trees may even be uprooted and fall on top of you.
- During the eye of the storm, move to the other side of your shelter, since the wind will now come from the opposite direction.
- After the winds die down, wait for at least 1½ hours before leaving your shelter.

HELPING CHILDREN COPE

Children may find a hurricane terrifying, especially if their home and belongings are damaged or if an evacuation is necessary. To help them feel more secure, try the following.

- Explain that a hurricane is a very bad storm and that the family might need to go to a safer building.
- Ask children to help you with simple tasks.

- Keep them occupied by taking activities such as cards into the safe room or hurricane shelter.
- Write each child's name, address, and contact number on a piece of paper and place it in the child's pocket.

Comforting children
Reassure young children and allay their fears by holding them and giving them plenty of attention.

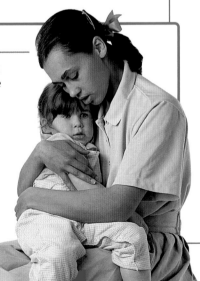

Tornado

◀ For **SEVERE STORM** see p.226 ▶ For **HURRICANE** see p.234

Tall columns of spinning air moving at high speeds are capable of causing immense damage. Tornadoes usually occur during warm, humid, unsettled weather but they can develop anywhere at any time, particularly after a thunderstorm or hurricane. If you live in a tornado area, make sure that you are familiar with the early warning system: a "tornado watch" indicates that a tornado is possible and a "tornado warning" means that a tornado has been seen and could be heading in your direction. Depending on the severity and path of the tornado, either stay under shelter or evacuate your home.

PREPARING FOR A TORNADO

1 Take precautions

- Keep alert for a "tornado watch" and listen to local radio stations for updates.
- Close hurricane shutters or board your windows (p.234) to protect yourself from flying glass (but see point 2 below).
- Choose a safe part of your house where family members can gather if a tornado is on the way (p.234, Take precautions).
- Fill clean baths, sinks, containers, and plastic bottles with water to ensure an uncontaminated supply.
- Fill your vehicle's tank with fuel.

2 Listen for warning

- If a "tornado watch" turns into a "tornado warning", be prepared to evacuate your home. If you are in a car, caravan, or mobile home, get out (see Stay safe, p.237).
- If warnings predict that your home will be in the tornado's direct path, open doors, shutters, and windows on the side away from the storm to prevent a build-up of air pressure.

3 Get to safety

- If you are told to evacuate, follow the instructions carefully.
- Act promptly, but calmly. You may have only a short time in which to get to the nearest hurricane shelter.

SIGNS AND WARNINGS

- Certain changes in weather conditions may herald a tornado, such as blowing debris or a sudden wind drop and unusually still air.
- In some circumstances, a low rumbling noise, the sound of an approaching tornado, may be audible.
- Tornadoes can be seen approaching, often from a great distance, moving at speeds of up to 50–60 km/h (30–40 mph).
- A tall funnel shape of whirling air and dust will descend from underneath a storm cloud.

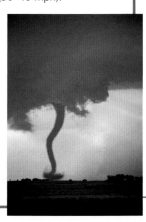

Violent tornado
The characteristic twisting funnel of air and dust indicates an approaching tornado.

DURING A TORNADO

1 Stay safe

- If a "tornado watch" turns into a "tornado warning" but you are advised not to evacuate, go to your chosen safe place in your house.
- Protect yourself and your family by crawling under a heavy piece of furniture, such as a table or desk.
- If you are unable to hide under furniture, sit down in the centre of the room and protect your head with your arms.
- If you are in a car, caravan, or mobile home, get out at once and head for open ground. Lay down flat and cover your head. Vehicles can be picked up by a forceful tornado and then dropped again, so they are not safe places in which to shelter.

2 Stay informed

- Listen to your radio for updated local information and official instructions. You may be asked to turn off utilities or to evacuate if the tornado alters course.
- If you are advised to evacuate, follow all instructions carefully.

3 Return home

- Once the tornado has passed, wait at least 5 minutes before leaving your place of shelter.

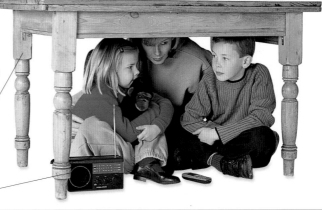

Choose a sturdy piece of furniture as your shelter

Take your radio with you to stay informed

! If you are outside

- Find the nearest sturdy building and head for the basement or lay down on the ground floor.
- If you are close to a bridge, get underneath it.
- If there is no obvious shelter, lay flat on the ground, away from trees or structures that could collapse, and ideally in a ditch. Cover your head with your hands.
- Be aware of the dangers of flying objects, falling trees, buildings that may collapse, and damaged power lines.

- If you are in a car, do not try to outdrive a tornado: if it changes course you will be in danger of being picked up in your vehicle.
- Get out of the car immediately and either find shelter or lay in a ditch or other low-lying land with your hands over your head.

Protecting yourself
If you are unable to locate a shelter, find a low-lying area and lay down, taking care to protect your head.

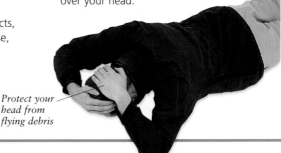

Protect your head from flying debris

Earthquake

◄ For **WILDFIRE** see p.232 ► For **TSUNAMI** see p.242

Earthquakes may strike without warning along fault lines, causing major damage and loss of life. Quakes often last for only seconds, but in that time buildings and roads can be destroyed and people crushed. Fires resulting from broken gas pipes can rage for days afterwards, and aftershocks are a further hazard. If you live in an earthquake area, prepare your home as best you can.

PREPARING FOR AN EARTHQUAKE

1 Identify potential hazards

- Check structural elements in your home (see p.222) to ensure that they are sound and see that heavy furniture is secure (see box below).
- Place large, heavy objects on lower shelves and rehang heavy mirrors or pictures that are currently positioned over seating or beds.
- Store fragile items in low cabinets that are fitted with latches or locks.

SECURING FURNITURE

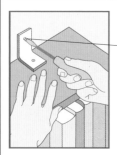

Screw the bracket into the wall and the bookcase

Attach furniture
Fit exterior angle brackets at the top or sides of tall furniture like bookcases and wardrobes

Use steel straps at top and bottom to secure the boiler to the wall

Secure boiler
Use galvanized steel straps, with holes punched through them, to attach a boiler to the wall

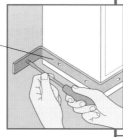

2 Identify safe places

- Identify safe spots in every room where you could take shelter. Ideal places are under a sturdy desk or table or beneath a strong internal doorway well away from windows, or where glass could shatter.
- Identify at least one safe outdoor location that you could escape to if necessary. Try to find a spot that is out in the open, well away from buildings, trees, power lines, and elevated roads and bridges, all of which are dangerous because they could fall or collapse.
- Make sure that every member of your family knows what to do in the event of an earthquake (p.239).

3 Be ready

- Be alert for small tremors, known as fore-shocks. These indicate that a larger earthquake is on its way. If you do feel a fore-shock, warn family members and head for a safe location at once.
- Be prepared to experience a ripple of after-shocks following the main earthquake. These after-shocks can also be severe and may cause additional damage.

DURING AN EARTHQUAKE

1 Take cover

- If you feel the ground shake, drop under a heavy desk or table, press your face against your arm to protect your eyes, and hold on.
- If you cannot reach a table, take shelter in an internal doorway.

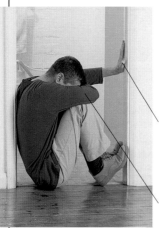

Brace yourself against a support

Cover your eyes with your arm

- If you cannot move quickly to a safe place, stay where you are but keep well away from windows.
- If you are in bed, stay there and protect your head with a pillow.
- Stay exactly where you are until the shaking stops.

2 Expect after-shocks

- Put out candles or naked flames in case of gas leaks. If you smell gas, turn off the supply at the mains.
- Each time you feel an after-shock, take cover and hold on, as before.
- Be aware that structures weakened by an earthquake can be toppled by after-shocks. Inspect your home for damage after each after-shock, and move everyone out of the building quickly if you suspect that it may be at all unsafe.

DO'S AND DON'TS

DO
- Keep away from windows: they could be shattered.
- Take cover wherever you are.
- Stay away from items that might fall on you, such as tall furniture.
- Put out cigarettes in case of gas leaks.

DON'T
- Use stairs or lifts.
- Run into the street: falling masonry or glass could injure you.
- Think that you are safe once the ground stops shaking: always expect after-shocks.
- Use telephones unless the call is essential.

---

3 Stay safe

- If you are inside and your home seems to be structurally sound, wait there until you are given the official all clear. Then prepare to leave and stay elsewhere until your home has been checked by a surveyor.
- Check everyone for injuries and give first-aid treatment as necessary.
- If water pipes are damaged, turn off your supply at the mains.
- If you can smell gas or suspect that electrical wiring is damaged, turn off supplies at the mains.
- Keep listening to your radio for official instructions.
- If you are outside, do not go back into your home until it has been checked for structural safety.

! If you are outside

- Lay down as far away as possible from buildings, trees, and power lines, or seek shelter in a doorway. Stay where you are until the shaking stops.
- Do not go into any form of underground shelter, such as a cellar or subway, because it could collapse.
- If you are driving, stop your car carefully and stay in your car until the shaking stops.

Volcanic eruption

◄ For EARTHQUAKE see p.238   ► For TSUNAMI see p.242

An erupting volcano sends clouds of ash billowing into the sky, rock fragments hurtling down to earth, and molten lava and mud flowing down its sides, often with little or no warning. You increase your chances of escaping unharmed if you leave the area as soon as you are advised to do so.

ESCAPING A VOLCANIC ERUPTION

① Be prepared

- If you live anywhere near a volcano, whether it is dormant or active, keep a pair of goggles and a disposable dust mask for each family member.

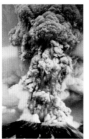

VOLCANO

- Make sure that you have planned at least two routes out of the area and arranged where to meet family members.

⚠ Warning signs

Professional vulcanologists study grumbling volcanoes for indications of increased activity. The following are all warning signs that a volcano might be about to erupt:

- An increase in seismic activity, ranging from minor tremors to earthquakes.
- Rumbling noises coming from the volcano.
- A cloud of steam hanging over the top of the volcano.
- A smell of sulphur from local rivers.
- Falls of acidic rain.
- Fine dust suspended in the sky.
- Occasional bursts of hot gases or ash from the volcano top.

② Evacuate

- If there is advance warning of an eruption, you may be advised to evacuate the area, in which case you should leave immediately.
- Make sure that you follow all the evacuation instructions carefully.
- To avoid your skin being irritated by ashfall, put on clothing that covers your entire body.
- Put on goggles and a disposable dust mask. If you do not have a mask, then improvise by wrapping either a wet scarf or a handkerchief around your face.

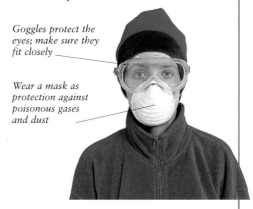

Goggles protect the eyes; make sure they fit closely

Wear a mask as protection against poisonous gases and dust

- Avoid areas that are downwind of the volcano because burning hot ash and clouds of gases may be blown in your direction.
- Avoid river valleys and low-lying areas, where mudflows may occur.

DURING A VOLCANIC ERUPTION

1 Follow instructions

- If a volcano erupts while you are at home, make sure that all family members and household pets are accounted for, and close all your doors, windows, and vents.
- If you are not advised to evacuate to the nearest emergency shelter, stay inside.
- Listen to your radio for official instructions. A period of calm may follow an eruption, so be prepared to leave to escape further eruptions if advised to do so.

! If you are outside

- Try to get inside a building.
- If you are caught in a rock fall, roll into a ball to protect your head.
- If you suspect that you are in the path of a nuée ardente (see box below), your only chances of survival are to shelter underground or to submerge yourself in water. The danger will usually have passed after just 30 seconds.
- If you are caught near a stream, beware of mudflows (see box below). Do not cross a bridge if a mudflow is moving beneath it because the bridge could be swept away.

2 Beware of ashfall

- If you have breathing problems, such as asthma, stay inside.
- Press damp towels firmly around doors and windows, and any other draught sources.
- Avoid driving: heavy ashfall clogs engines, which can stall cars.
- Clear volcanic ash from the roof of your house: its weight can cause buildings to collapse. Be careful when working on the roof, and put on protective clothing, goggles, and a dust mask before going out.

3 Stay safe

- If you were evacuated, stay out of any restricted areas until you are given the official all-clear.
- Be aware that mudflows, ashfall, flash floods, and wildfires can reach you even if you are far from the volcano and are unable to see it.
- When you return home, or if you remained there, dampen and clean up ash that has settled around the house, being careful not to wash it into drains. Put on your protective clothing, goggles, and a dust mask.

UNDERSTANDING THE DANGERS

- Ash and other debris rain down from the sky, covering buildings, land, and people.
- Debris flows are a mixture of water and volcanic debris that flows down the volcano sides. They can travel long distances and destroy whole villages.
- Mudflows are fast-moving rivers of mud that flow from volcanoes down river valleys and over low-lying areas.

- Lava flows are fairly unlikely to kill you because they move slowly, but anything that stands in their path will be burned, crushed, or buried.
- Pyroclastic surges are mixtures of rock fragments and hot gases that move rapidly across land like a hurricane. Anyone who is caught in their path is likely to be either burned, asphyxiated, or crushed.

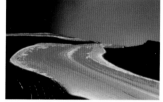

RED-HOT LAVA FLOW

- Nuées ardentes are rapidly moving, red-hot clouds of ash, gas, and rock fragments that flow down the side of a volcano at speeds of over 160 km/h (100 mph).

Tsunami

◀ For FLOOD see p.228   ◀ For EARTHQUAKE see p.238
An earthquake, volcanic eruption, or underwater landslide can cause a tsunami: a series of underwater waves that sweep towards shore, sometimes rising to heights of over 30 m (100 ft), and causing immense damage. A "tsunami advisory" means that a tsunami is possible; a "tsunami watch" is issued when a tsunami may be 2 hours away; and a "tsunami warning" means that giant waves may be imminent. If you live within 3.2 km (2 miles) of the shore and your house is below 30 m (100 ft) above sea level, evacuate on receiving a "tsunami warning" and move to high ground as far inland as you can go.

PREPARING FOR A TSUNAMI

1 Be aware

- Keep alert for a "tsunami advisory" or "tsunami watch" and listen to local radio stations for updates.
- Check that your planned escape route is clear.
- Familiarize yourself with warning signs, such as a sudden change in the level of coastal waters.
- Tsunamis often cause severe floods; make sure that you are prepared to cope (p.228).

2 Take precautions

- Keep your car filled with fuel so that you can drive to safety at a moment's notice.
- If a "tsunami watch" turns into an "tsunami warning", prepare to evacuate your home.
- Coastal areas within 1.6 km (1 mile) of the sea and less than 7.5 m (25 ft) above sea level are most at risk; make an early assessment of the best route to higher ground.

UNDERSTANDING TSUNAMIS

- Earthquakes, underwater landslides, or volcanic eruptions can cause tsunamis.
- Each tsunami consists of a series of waves travelling at speeds of up to 970 km/h (600 mph).
- These waves are hundreds of kilometres (miles) long but only a metre or so (a few feet) "tall" as they travel the ocean floor. This means that they cannot be detected from the air or by shipping until they near the shore.
- Seismic activity may be the only advance warning of an approaching tsunami.
- As the tsunami nears the coast, the waves slow down and increase in height.
- Before the first wave reaches the shore, the sea may be dramatically "sucked" away from the shoreline.
- Successive waves appear at intervals of 5 to 90 minutes.
- The first wave is usually not the largest; the following ones cause the most damage.

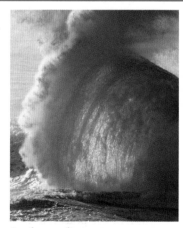

Sea-borne disaster
Vast sea waves crash on to the shore, causing damage and claiming lives.

DURING A TSUNAMI

1 Get to safety

- If you are advised to evacuate, follow all instructions carefully and leave as quickly as possible.
- Go to your planned evacuation place or follow instructions for a recommended evacuation route, if issued. Your place of safety should be at least 30 m (100 ft) above sea level or 3.2 km (2 miles) inland.

2 Stay informed

- Keep listening to your radio for updated local information and official instructions.
- Stay on high ground and inland until the official all-clear is given.

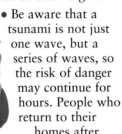

- Be aware that a tsunami is not just one wave, but a series of waves, so the risk of danger may continue for hours. People who return to their homes after the first wave (often not the biggest) risk being drowned.

3 Check damage

- When you are allowed to return to your home, inspect the structure of the building carefully for cracks or weaknesses. Tsunami waters often damage foundations and walls.
- Enter cautiously because there may be hazards hidden under the water.
- Check for potential fire hazards, such as broken gas pipes or flooded electrical circuits.

! If you feel an earthquake on the coast

- Drop to the ground, crawl to a sturdy shelter, if possible, and put your hands over your head to protect it.
- When the shaking stops, gather your family and evacuate; move inland and to higher ground as quickly as possible: a tsunami may be only minutes away.
- Stay away from any structures that may have been weakened by the earthquake.
- Do not leave your place of safety until an official all-clear has been issued.

4 Stay safe

- Do not use tap water unless you have been officially advised that it is safe to do so.
- Open doors and windows to help the building dry out.
- Inspect all your food and drink supplies and throw away any items that are wet.
- If you smell gas, turn off the supply at the mains, open your doors and windows, and leave at once.
- If electrical wiring has become wet or damaged, turn off the electricity supply at the mains.

DO'S AND DON'TS

DO	DON'T
• Go as far inland and as high as you can to escape the water.	• Try to watch the giant waves come ashore.
• Be careful on returning home: the tsunami may have caused structural damage.	• Leave your place of safety after the first wave: wait for the official all-clear before returning home.
• Use bottled water until you are told that tap water is safe.	• Enter your home with a naked flame: there may be a gas leak.

Post-disaster survival

Once a severe natural disaster is over, life may not return to normal for some time; in the case of an earthquake or volcanic eruption, it may be weeks before normal life resumes. In the meantime, keep out of danger, find temporary shelter, if necessary, and conserve food and water supplies. Check your home for damage, and find temporary accommodation if you suspect that it may be unsound.

ACTION PLAN

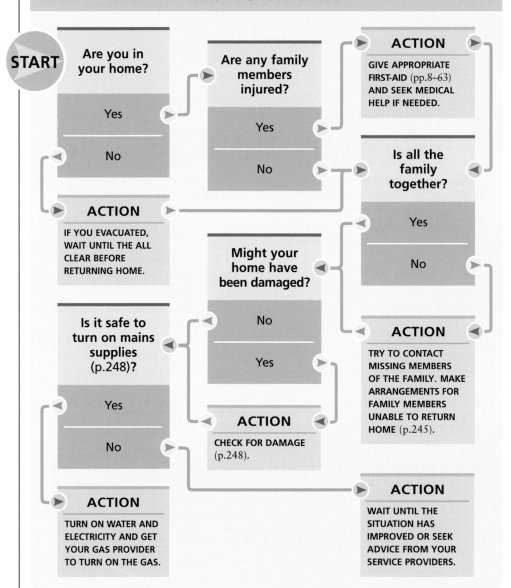

START

Are you in your home?
- Yes
- No

ACTION
IF YOU EVACUATED, WAIT UNTIL THE ALL CLEAR BEFORE RETURNING HOME.

Are any family members injured?
- Yes
- No

ACTION
GIVE APPROPRIATE FIRST-AID (pp.8–63) AND SEEK MEDICAL HELP IF NEEDED.

Is all the family together?
- Yes
- No

ACTION
TRY TO CONTACT MISSING MEMBERS OF THE FAMILY. MAKE ARRANGEMENTS FOR FAMILY MEMBERS UNABLE TO RETURN HOME (p.245).

Might your home have been damaged?
- No
- Yes

ACTION
CHECK FOR DAMAGE (p.248).

Is it safe to turn on mains supplies (p.248)?
- Yes
- No

ACTION
TURN ON WATER AND ELECTRICITY AND GET YOUR GAS PROVIDER TO TURN ON THE GAS.

ACTION
WAIT UNTIL THE SITUATION HAS IMPROVED OR SEEK ADVICE FROM YOUR SERVICE PROVIDERS.

IMMEDIATE AFTERMATH

1 Assess situation

- If the disaster was severe but you remained in your home, you will usually be advised to stay there unless you think that the building is structurally unsound.
- You are generally safer in your home, away from external dangers, and by staying inside you will not obstruct the emergency services.
- Assess your home for minor damage, some of which you may be able to repair, and for the safety of mains supplies (p.248).
- Listen to your radio or watch television (if you have electricity) to assess the scale of the disaster and its aftermath.
- If the incident had minor, or no effects on your home and family, resume your daily activities as normal, but be aware that nearby areas may have been more seriously affected and could be dangerous.

2 Treat injuries

- If any members of the family have been injured during the disaster, give them appropriate first-aid treatment (pp.8–63). Always seek medical help if injuries are severe.

3 Make contact

- If you have been separated from family members who were unable to shelter in the house with you, you will want to make contact as soon as possible.
- Try to get in touch by mobile phone or call the friend or relative at the second emergency meeting place in your disaster plan (p.223).
- Keep calls to a minimum to avoid blocking lines badly needed by the emergency services.
- If you can move around safely in the local area, visit neighbours, especially, the elderly or disabled, to see if they need help or supplies.
- If you were not at home when the disaster struck, contact family members as soon as possible to reassure them that you are safe.

4 Try to reach help

- If you or your family were not at home and cannot now reach either home, your second meeting place, or an evacuation shelter, you may have to survive outside until you can reach help. (See pp.246–7 for advice on surviving outside.)

DEALING WITH STRANDED FAMILY MEMBERS

- If the disaster has caused damage, such as roads blocked by fallen trees or flooding, school children may not be able to return home that evening. Ask a friend to collect them and keep them for the night.
- If the situation is severe, you may need to make arrangements for your children for a few days until travel is possible.
- If you cannot make contact with your stranded children for any reason, ask the emergency services for their help.
- Family members working outside the immediate area may also be stranded and unable to return home. They will need to make alternative accommodation arrangements until the situation improves.

SURVIVING OUTSIDE

1 Avoid danger

- Any post-disaster area will be full of potential hazards, so stay alert and move around carefully.
- Keep well away from damaged power lines: high-voltage electricity is very dangerous and can cause electrocution and fire.
- Leaking gas pipes are also a danger. If you smell gas, you should leave the area immediately.
- If sewage pipes are damaged, there is the risk that raw sewage could spill out in the open, leading to the rapid spread of disease.
- Buildings that become unstable following a natural disaster could topple at any time. Keep away from tall buildings and structures.

! Heat exposure

- Prolonged exposure to strong sunlight can lead to illness as a result of sunburn (p.50), heat exhaustion (p.51), and/or heatstroke (p.52).
- For all these conditions, the first step is to move the person to a cool place.
- Cool sunburned skin with cold water and give the person cold drinks to sip.
- Symptoms of heat exhaustion are headache, dizziness, nausea, and rapid pulse. Give the person an isotonic drink or a weak salt and sugar solution (p.51).
- Symptoms of heatstroke are headache, dizziness, flushed skin, and, in serious cases, unconsciousness. Remove the person's outer clothing, lay him or her down, then cool the skin by repeatedly sponging cold water over it.

! Cold exposure

- If the weather is very cold and you do not manage to find shelter, you are at risk of developing frostbite (p.55) and/or hypothermia (p.54).
- Symptoms of frostbite include "pins-and-needles", followed by numbness. Skin may be white, mottled and blue, or black.
- Symptoms of hypothermia include very cold skin, shivering, apathy, poor vision, and irritable behaviour.
- For either condition, put the person into a sleeping bag or wrap in a survival blanket (covering the head too). Frostbitten fingers may be tucked under the armpits for extra warmth. Give warm sweet drinks.

Keeping warm
Wrap the person in a survival blanket, and cover her head if she is not wearing a hat.

2 Find shelter

- If you had to evacuate your home but did not manage to reach either your chosen place of evacuation or a local emergency shelter, you will need to find some form of shelter for your family.
- If you are in a town, try to find an empty building in which you could take shelter. Avoid buildings that look as though they may be structurally unsound, especially following an earthquake.
- If you are in the countryside, look for either a manmade structure, such as a bridge, a barn or a shed. As a last resort, trees will at least protect you from extremes of temperature, wind, rain, or snow.
- Use the bedding supplies in your disaster emergency kit (p.225) to keep you warm at night.

3 Create shelter

- If you cannot find shelter, try to build one from any materials you may find to hand.
- You need to build a structure that will provide adequate protection from the wind, rain, and sun.
- If you are in the countryside, you could use vegetation and branches to construct a lean-to shelter.
- If you are in a town, hunt around for sheets of metal, plastic sheeting, pieces of wood, or anything else you can find that could be used to create a shelter.
- Involve all family members in constructing the shelter. Not only will the work be done more quickly, but it will keep you all occupied.

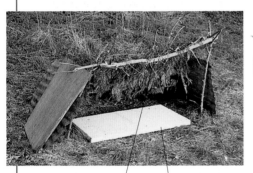

Make a roof out of vegetation strapped to a wooden frame

Find something water-resistant to use as a floor

4 Keep positive

- Unpack your disaster emergency kit and find places for everyone to spread out their sleeping bags. Make your shelter as comfortable as possible.
- Comfort young children by telling them how exciting your "camping" experience will be.
- Try to keep up morale with the thought that you are all safe and that this is only a temporary situation until help arrives.

5 Build fire

- If it is cold, build a fire. If you are in the countryside, use twigs and small branches, but be aware of the dangers of starting a wildfire. If you are in a town, use whatever materials are available.
- If you have suitable containers with you, you may be able to heat up some of your emergency food.

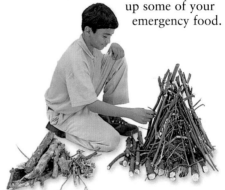

6 Conserve food and water

- If you are unable to reach safety or help fails to arrive within 2 days, think about conserving your supplies of food and water.
- Restrict adult rations but give children, the elderly, and pregnant women normal supplies, if possible.
- Be aware that water is more vital than food: a healthy adult can survive without food for a week with no serious health effects, but more than 1–2 days without water can be highly dangerous.
- If water supplies run low, collect rainfall to drink.
- Alternatively, find the cleanest-looking source you can and purify it to make it drinkable (p.249).
- Do not drink water from streams or damaged pipes: it could be contaminated and could seriously damage your health.

CHECKING YOUR HOME

1 Check for damage

- Do not enter your home if there is water around it. Flood water can undermine foundations, causing buildings to sink, floors to crack, or walls to collapse.
- Check the outside of your home for signs of structural damage, such as cracks in walls, a leaning chimney, and walls at angles.
- If you are certain that it is safe to enter your home, go inside and inspect the walls, floors, windows, doors, and staircases for damage.
- Do not enter your home carrying any naked flame, such a lighted cigarette, in case of gas leaks.
- If in any doubt, ask a structural engineer to inspect your home.

2 Check safety of mains supplies

- If you remained in your house and did not turn off mains supplies, be aware of the possible dangers.
- If wiring has been damaged, turn off electricity at the mains and ask an electrician to inspect it.
- If you can smell gas, turn off the supply at the mains, open doors and windows, and leave at once.
- If sewage pipes are damaged, shut off your water supply at the mains stopcock (outside your house). This will prevent contaminated water entering your water system.
- Do not drink tap water unless you have been officially told it is safe.
- If you turned off mains supplies before the disaster, and are certain that they are safe, turn on the water and electricity, and ask your gas supplier to turn on the gas.

3 Make repairs

- Check for minor damage in your home, such as cracked or missing roof tiles and leaks. Remedy any problems as quickly as possible, using short-term measures, if necessary, until proper repair work can be undertaken.
- If your home has been shaken by the disaster, causing breakages and spillages, clean up dangerous debris as quickly as possible. Shattered glass and spilled flammable liquids and bleaches can all be potentially extremely dangerous.

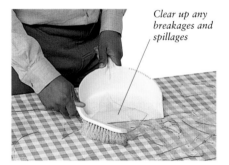

Clear up any breakages and spillages

4 Contact your insurance company

- Call your insurance company's emergency helpline as soon as possible. You will be given advice on what to do.
- If immediate repairs are necessary, arrange for them to be carried out straight away. Keep the receipts to give to your insurers later.
- Your insurance company will send a loss adjuster to assess extensive damage and the cost of reparation.
- Take photographs or videos of the damage to corroborate insurance claims and keep copies of all your correspondence with insurers.

LOOKING AFTER YOUR FAMILY

1 Cope with power loss

- You may have to cope without supplies of gas and electricity for a period of time, particularly if the disaster has been serious enough to affect the local infrastructure.
- Use torches or candles at night, but conserve supplies by using them only if absolutely necessary.
- If you have a working hearth and chimney, forage for wood to burn, but be aware of the danger of chimney fires in a dirty chimney.

2 Use food sensibly

- Without electricity to power fridges and freezers, chilled or frozen foods will soon become inedible.
- Avoid opening fridge and freezer doors too often in order to conserve the cold air inside.
- A fully stocked, well-insulated freezer should keep foods frozen for at least 3 days, so use supplies from the fridge first. Only foods that do not require cooking will be usable, unless you have a camping stove.
- Once these supplies are finished, turn to stores of canned and dried foods.

3 Keep up morale

- The aftermath of a major natural disaster will be a difficult period. Family members or friends may be unaccounted for, you may have to cope with injuries, and there will almost certainly be damage and suffering all around.
- Help your family to remain positive and keep them focused on the issue of surviving. Keep busy and try to work together as a team, making sure that you discuss any plans.
- Reassure young children that you have survived and that the worst is over. Keep them entertained to distract them from the situation.
- Bear in mind the comfort factor of food. In a time of great stress and upheaval, a familiar food or drink can be very reassuring.

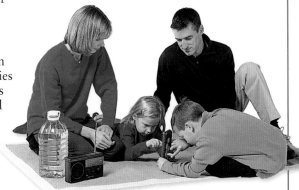

PURIFYING WATER

If water supplies run low and mains water is contaminated, you will have to purify water.

- If you can see particles floating in water, strain it through some paper towels then boil it, add purifying tablets, or disinfect it.
- Boil some water for 10 minutes to purify it, then allow it to cool before drinking.
- Use chlorine-based tablets to purify water.

- To disinfect water, use regular household bleach containing 5.25 per cent sodium hypochlorite only. A stronger percentage is dangerous.
- Add two drops of bleach to 500 ml (1 pt) of water, stir and leave it to stand for 30 minutes. The water should smell slightly of bleach. If it does not, repeat the process and leave the water to stand for a further 15 minutes.

Useful online sites and addresses

FIRST-AID ORGANIZATIONS

British Red Cross
9 Grosvenor Crescent
London SW1X 7EJ
Tel: (020) 7235 5454
Online: www.redcross.org.uk

St Andrew's Ambulance Association
St Andrew's House
48 Milton Street
Glasgow G4 OHR
Tel: (0141) 332 4031
Online: www.firstaid.org.uk

St John Ambulance
1 Grosvenor Crescent
London SW1X 7EF
Tel: 08700 10 49 50
Online: www.sja.org.uk

DIY HELP

Gas Emergency
Freephone: 0800 111 999

House.co.uk
Advice on problems around the home
Online: www.house.co.uk

Royal Society for the Prevention of Accidents
RoSPA
Edgbaston Park
353 Bristol Road
Edgbaston
Birmingham B5 7ST
Tel: (0121) 248 2000
E-mail: help@rospa.co.uk
Online: www.rospa.co.uk

GENERAL HEALTHCARE

BBC Online Health and Fitness
Online: www.bbc.co.uk/health

British Medical Association
BMA House
Tavistock Square
London WC1H 9JP
Tel: (0205) 7387 4499
E-mail: info.web@bma.org.uk
Online: www.bma.org.uk

Foundation for Women's Health Research and Development
40 Eastbourne Terrace
London W2 6LX
Tel: (020) 7725 2606
Online: www.forwarddircon.co.uk

Healthnet
Heart care information
Online: www.healthnet.org.uk

Help the Aged
207–221 Pentonville Road
London N1 9UZ
Tel: (020) 7278 1114
E-mail: info@helptheaged.org.uk
Online: www.helptheaged.org.uk

NetDoctor
UK-based independent health website
Online: www.netdoctor.co.uk

NHS Direct
Helpline for health problems with links to other sites
Helpline: 0845 4647
Online: www.nhsdirect.nhs.uk

Patient UK
Directory of websites providing information on health issues
E-mail: info@patient.co.uk
Online: www.patient.co.uk

ParentsTalk
Advice on family health
Online: www.parents-talk.com

UK Homeopathic Medical Association
6 Livingstone Road
Gravesend
Kent DA12 5D2
Tel: (01474) 560336
E-mail: info@the-hma.org
Online: www.the-hma.org

MASTER TRADESMEN

Federation of Master Builders
14 Great James Street
London WC1 N 3DP
Tel: (020) 7242 7583
Online: www.fmb.org.uk

Master Locksmiths Association
Unit 5D
Great Central Way
Woodford House
Daventry NN11 3PZ
Tel: (01327) 262255
Online: www.locksmiths.co.uk

NATURAL DISASTERS

American Red Cross
Provides detailed information on how to prepare for and survive natural disasters
Online: www.redcross.org

Earthquake and forensic seismology and geomagnetism programme
British Geological Survey
Murchison House
West Mains Road
Edinburgh EH9 3LA
Tel: (0131) 667 1000

Earthquake and other queries
E-mail: ukeqs@bgs.ac.uk
Online: www.gsgr.nmh.ac.uk

Environment Agency
Rio House
Waterside Drive
Aztec West, Almondsbury
Bristol BS32 4UD
Tel: 0845 933 3111
E-mail: enquiries@ environment-agency.gov.uk
Online: www.environment-agency.gov.uk/flood
Floodline – flood warnings, and 24-hour advice and information on floods.
Tel: 0845 988 1188

Federal Emergency Management Agency
US site providing information on preparedness
Online: www.fema.gov

Online Weather
Worldwide weather forecasts
Online: www.onlineweather.com

Survivaldisaster.com
Survival information and tips
Online: www.survivaldisaster.com

The Geological Society
Burlington House
Piccadilly
London W1J OBG
Tel: (020) 7434 9944
E-mail: enquiries@geolsoc.org.uk
Online: www.geolsoc.org.uk

The Global Earthquake Response Center
Online: www.earthquake.com

Tornado and Storm Research Organization
British-based independent and privately supported research body, serving the European public interest.
Online: www.torro.org.uk

HOME SECURITY

National Association of Victim Support Schemes
Cranmer House
39 Brixton Road
London SW9 6D2
Helpline: 0845 3030 9000
Tel: (020) 7735 9166
Online: www.victimsupport.org

National Neighbourhood Watch Association
Schomberg House
80-82 Pall Mall
London SW1Y 5HF
Tel: (020) 7772 3348
Online: www.neighbourhoodwatch.net

The Burgled Helpline
Online: www.burgled.com

SPECIFIC HEALTH PROBLEMS

BackCare
16 Elmtree Road
Teddington
Middlesex TW11 86T
Tel: (020) 8977 5474
Online: www.backpain.org

Breast Cancer Care
210 New Kings Road
London SW6 4NZ
Helpline: 0808 800 6000
Tel: (020) 7384 2984
E-mail: bcc@breastcancercare.org.uk
Online: www.breastcancercare.org.uk

British Allergy Foundation
30 Bellegrove Road
Welling, Kent DA16 3PY
Helpline: (020) 8303 8583
Tel: (020) 8303 8525
E-mail: info@allergyfoundation.com
Online: www.allergyfoundation.com

British Association of Dermatologists
19 Fitzroy Square
London WC1
Tel: (020) 7383 0266
E-mail: admin@bad.org.uk
Online: www.bad.org.uk

British Brain and Spine Foundation
7 Winchester House
Kennington Park
Cranmer Road
London SW9 6EJ
Helpline: 0808 808 1000
Tel: (020) 7793 5900
Online: www.bbsf.org.uk

British Diabetic Association
10 Queen Anne Street
London W1G 9LH
Tel: (020) 7323 1531
E-mail: info@diabetes.org.uk
Online: www.diabetes.org.uk

British Digestive Foundation
3 St Andrews Place
London NW1 4LS
Tel: (020) 7486 0341
Online: www.digestivedisorders.org.uk

British Epilepsy Association
New Anstey House
Gate Way Drive
Yeadon, Leeds
LS19 7XY
Helpline: 0808 800 5050
Tel: (0013) 210 8800
E-mail: epilepsy@epilepsy.org.uk
Online: www.epilepsy.org.uk

British Heart Foundation
14 Fitzhardinge Street
London W1H 4DH
Heartline: 0990 200656
Tel: (020) 7935 0185
E-mail: internet@bhf.org.uk
Online: www.bhf.org.uk

British Lung Foundation
78 Hatton Garden
London EC1N 8LD
Tel: (020) 7831 5831
E-mail: blf@british lungfoundation.com
Online: www.lunguk.org

Headway (National Head Injuries Association)
7 King Edward Court
King Edward Street
Nottingham NG1 1EW
Tel: (0115) 924 0800
E-mail: information@headway.org.uk
Online: www.headway.org.uk

Hyperhydrosis
Help with profuse sweating
Online: www.excessivesweating.org

Incontact – Action on Incontinence
United House, North Road
London N7 8DP
Tel (020) 7700 7035
E-mail: info@incontact.org
Online: www.incontact.org

Interstitital Cystitis Support Group
76 High Street, Stony Stratford
Bucks MK 11 1AH
Tel: (01908) 569169
E-mail: info@interstitialcystitis.co.uk
Online: www.interstitialcystitis.co.uk

Irritable Bowel Syndrome Network (IBS Network)
Northern General Hospital
Sheffield S5 7AU
E-mail:
penny@ibsnetwork.org.uk
Online: www.ibsnetwork.org.uk

Migraine Action Association
Unit 6 Oakley Hay Lodge
Business Park
Great Folds Road
Great Oakley
Northants NN18 9AS
Tel: (01536) 461333
E-mail: info@migraine.org.uk
Online: www.migraine.org.uk

Moorfields Eye Hospital
162 City Road
London EC1V 8PD
Tel: (020) 7253 3411
Helpline: (020) 7566 2345
Online: www.moorfields.org.uk

National Association for Colitis and Crohn's Disease
4 Beaumont House
Sutton Road
St Albans
Hertfordshire AL1 5HH
Tel: (01727) 844296
E-mail: nacc@nacc.org.uk
Online: www.nacc.org.uk

National Asthma Campaign
Providence House
Providence Place
London N1 ONT
Helpline: 0845 701 0203
Tel: (020) 7226 2260
Online: www.asthma.org.uk

National Eczema Society
Hill House
Highgate Hill
London N19 5NA
Helpline: 0870 241 3604
Tel: (020) 7281 3553
Online: www.eczema.org

National Endometriosis Society
50 Westminster Palace Gardens
Artillery Row
London SW1P 1RL
Freephone: 0808 808 2227
Helpline: (020) 7222 2781
Online: www.endo.org.uk

National Meningitis Trust
Fern House
Bath Road, Stroud
24-hr support: 0845 600 0800
Online:
www.meningitis-trust.org.uk

Prostate Cancer Charity
3 Angel Walk
London W6 5HX
Confidential helpline:
0845 300 8383
Tel: (020) 8222 7622
E-mail:
info@prostate-cancer.org.uk
Online:
www.prostate-cancer.org.uk

The Alzheimer's Society
Gordon House
10 Greencoat Place
London SW1P 1PH
Tel: (020) 7306 0606
E-mail: info@alzheimers.org.uk
Online: www.alzheimers.org.uk

The Impotence Association
PO Box 10296
London SW17 9WH
Helpline: (020) 8767 7791
E-mail: thei@btinternet.com
Online: www.impotence.org.uk

The Stroke Association
123 Whitecross Street
London EC1Y 8JJ
Helpline: 0845 303 3100
Tel: (020) 7566 0300
Online: www.stroke.org.uk

TRADE ASSOCIATIONS

British Pest Control Association
1 Gleneagles House
Vernon Gate
South Street
Derby DE1 1UP
Tel: (01332) 294288
Online: www.bpca.org.uk

British Security Industry Association
Security House
Barbourne Road
Worcester WR1 1RS
Tel: (01905) 21464
Online: www.bsia.co.uk

British Wood Preserving and Damp Proofing Association
1 Gleneagles House
Vernon Gate, South Street
Derby DE1 1UP
Tel: (01332) 225100
Online: www.bwpda.co.uk

Glass and Glazing Federation
44–48 Borough High Street
London SE1 1XB
Tel: (020) 7403 7177
Online: www.ggf.org.uk

Heating and Ventilating Contractors Association
Esca House, 34 Palace Court
London W2 4JG
Tel: (020) 7313 4900
Online: www.hvca.org.uk

Institute of Plumbing
64 Station Lane
Hornchurch
Essex RM12 6NB
Tel: (01708) 474791
Online: www.plumbers.org.uk

National Federation of Roofing Contractors
24 Weymouth Street
London W1G 7LX
Tel: (020) 7436 0387
Online: www.nfrc.co.uk

National Inspection Council for Electrical Installation Contracting
37 Albert Embankment
London SE1 7UJ
Tel: (020) 7582 7746
Online: www.niceic.org.uk

TRAVEL ADVICE

Travel Advice Unit
Consular Division
Foreign and
Commonwealth Office
Old Admiralty Building
London SW1A 2PA
Tel: (020) 7008 0232/0233
E-mail:
consular.fco@gtnet.gov.uk
Online: www.fco.gov.uk

World Travel Guide
Online: www.travel-guide.com

Index

Acknowledgments

Cooling Brown would like to thank Derek Coombes, Elaine Hewson, and Elly King for design assistance, Kate Sheppard for editorial assistance, Dennis Fell for advice on air conditioning, and G. R. Coleman.

Dorling Kindersley would like to thank Andrea Bagg and Martyn Page for their editorial help, and Franziska Marking for picture research.

MODELS
Philip Argent, Flora Bendall, Imogen Bendall, Jennifer Bendall, Ross Bendall, Alison Bolus, Eleanor Bolus, Dale Buckton, Angela Cameron, Madeleine Cameron, Shenton Dickson, Olivia King, Michel Labat, Janey Madlani, Tish Mills

INDEX
Patricia Coward

ILLUSTRATORS
David Ashby, Kuo Kang Chen, Peter Cooling, Chris King, Patrick Mulrey, John Woodcock

PHOTOGRAPHERS
Matthew Ward, Trish Grant

PICTURE CREDITS
Colin Walton 210b, Corbis 236, Photodisc 240, 241, 242

JACKET PICTURE CREDITS
Pictor International front bl, front br; **Popperfoto** front bc; **Science Photo Library** BSIP, Laurent front tr; **Stone/Getty Images** back tc, back tl, front tc, front tl, spine.

All other images © Dorling Kindersley. For further information see: **www.dkimages.com**

EMERGENCY CONTACTS

- In the event of an emergency go to the nearest telephone and dial 999
- Ask for the police, ambulance or fire brigade

In case of an emergency please call

Name...
Telephone...
Mobile...

Relative

Name ....
Address...
....
Telephone ....
Mobile ....

Neighbour

Name ....
Address...
....
Telephone ....
Mobile ....

School

Name ....
Address...
....
Telephone ....

School

Name ....
Address...
....
Telephone ....

Place of work

Name ....
Address..
....
Telephone ....

Taxi service

Name ....
Telephone ....

Local police station

Address..
....
Telephone ....

Landlord

Name ....
Telephone ....

Intruder alarm company

Name ....
Address..
....
Telephone ....